VITAMIN A

**Everything
You Need
to Know**

Other Books From the People's Medical Society

Arthritis: Questions You Have . . . Answers You Need

Cholesterol and Triglycerides: Questions You Have . . . Answers You Need

Prostate: Questions You Have . . . Answers You Need

Stroke: Questions You Have . . . Answers You Need

Vitamin C: Everything You Need to Know

Vitamin E: Everything You Need to Know

Vitamins and Minerals: Questions You Have . . . Answers You Need

Your Eyes: Questions You Have . . . Answers You Need

Your Heart: Questions You Have . . . Answers You Need

VITAMIN A

Everything You Need to Know

By Janet Benton

People's Medical Society®

Allentown, Pennsylvania

The People's Medical Society is a nonprofit consumer health organization dedicated to the principles of better, more responsive and less expensive medical care. Organized in 1983, the People's Medical Society puts previously unavailable medical information into the hands of consumers so that they can make informed decisions about their own health care.

Membership in the People's Medical Society is $20 a year and includes a subscription to the *People's Medical Society Newsletter.* For information, write to the People's Medical Society, 462 Walnut Street, Allentown, PA 18102, or call 610-770-1670.

This and other People's Medical Society publications are available for quantity purchase at discount. Contact the People's Medical Society for details.

© 1998 by the People's Medical Society
Printed in the United States of America

Library of Congress Cataloging-in-Publication Data
Benton, Janet.
    Vitamin A : everything you need to know / by Janet Benton.
      p. cm.
    Includes index.
    ISBN 1-882606-44-2
    1. Vitamin A—Popular works. I. Title.
QP772.V5B46 1998
613.2'86—dc21   98-36550
                                                       CIP

1 2 3 4 5 6 7 8 9 0
First printing, October 1998

CONTENTS

Introduction 7

Chapter 1   The Basics 11

Chapter 2   Vitamin A and Carotenoids and Their Uses 31

Vitamin A and Carotenoids and the
Immune System 36

*Vitamin A and Carotenoids and
Immune Response* 37

Vitamin A and Carotenoids and Cancer 42

Vitamin A and Carotenoids and Cancer Risk . . 43

Lung Cancer 44

Breast Cancer 51

Colorectal Cancer 54

Liver Cancer 56

Prostate Cancer 56

Skin Cancer 58

Vitamin A and Carotenoids and
Cancer Treatment 59

Cancer-Fighting Mechanisms of
Vitamin A and Carotenoids 62

Vitamin A and Carotenoids and the
Cardiovascular System 65

*Vitamin A and Carotenoids and
Heart Disease* 66

*Heart-Protective Mechanisms of
Carotenoids* 74

Vitamin A and Carotenoids and the
Respiratory System 76

Vitamin A and Carotenoids and Smoking 77

Vitamin A and Carotenoids and Lung Disease. . 78

Vitamin A and Carotenoids and the Eyes 80

Vitamin A and Carotenoids and the Skin 82

Other Vitamin A and Carotenoid Uses 84

*Vitamin A and Carotenoids and
Human Immunodeficiency Virus* 84

Carotenoids and Rheumatoid Arthritis 87

Vitamin A and Premature Infants 88

Putting It All Together 89

Chapter 3 What Else Do I Need to Know? 91

Dosage 92

Toxicity 99

Drug Interactions 101

Nutrient Interactions 102

Supplements 103

Dietary Sources 107

Glossary 111

Index 119

INTRODUCTION

My mother always told me to eat my carrots if I wanted better vision. Of course, as a kid I did not know why carrots would help me see better, nor was I sure my mother's command was truthful (I suspected it might have been a ploy to get me to eat a vegetable I did not particularly like). Nevertheless, dutifully, if not reluctantly, I did eat my carrots, and now that I am well into middle age and still do not need glasses, I'm glad I did.

Obviously, 40 or more years ago, I did not know what carrots had in them that promoted strong vision, and I suspect that most other people did not either. But over the years, we have learned that carrots are rich in beta carotene, a carotenoid the body converts to vitamin A. And vitamin A, we've discovered, is key in the development of eye tissue and vision in children. It helps us see at night. And older folks who have had a diet rich in carotenoids (many of which can be converted to vitamin A) are less likely to develop macular degeneration—the number one cause of blindness in people over age 65.

But we have learned a lot more about this amazing vitamin and its carotenoid precursors. There is strong evidence that vitamin A enhances the body's immune system—helping it to fight off infection. Vitamin A is important for the skin, and carotenoids have been linked to helping lower cholesterol. And a number of studies suggest vitamin A and carotenoids may be significant ingredients in cancer prevention.

Yet as much as we know about vitamin A and carotenoids, it is hard to separate the facts from the hype. From less-than-scrupulous sales clerks to misleading advertisements, we are bombarded with claim upon claim about the wonders of vitamin A and carotenoids. And sadly, evidence cannot support many of those claims.

Which is why we have written this book. We felt it was time someone scoured the scientific studies about vitamin A and carotenoids with the express purpose of presenting the facts. And scour we did. What you will find in the pages that follow is the latest research on vitamin A and carotenoids. We tell you not only what these nutrients can do but also how they do it. We explain the best sources of vitamin A and carotenoids and how much a person needs each day. In other words, what you will learn from this book is everything you need to know about vitamin A and carotenoids—and you will learn it in an easy-to-read, easy-to-understand format.

For more than 15 years, the nonprofit People's Medical Society has been the nation's foremost source of consumer health information. In our more than 80 books and other health publications, we have presented health care consumers with the most vital information necessary to making health care decisions. Almost 4 million copies of our books have been sold, and consumers regularly tell us how helpful these books have been. That is why I am confident this book will be an invaluable resource to you.

CHARLES B. INLANDER
President
People's Medical Society

VITAMIN A

**Everything
You Need
to Know**

1 THE BASICS

Q: What is **vitamin A?**

A: Vitamin A is an essential **nutrient**, a substance necessary for survival that we must take in through diet and/or supplementation. In its **retinol** form, vitamin A is a clear yellow oil. Retinol is present naturally in butter, egg yolks, cream and milk, as well as in fish liver (and fish liver oils), beef liver and chicken liver. Liver is especially rich in the **vitamin**. Vitamin A is also an added nutrient in some fortified foods, including many low-fat milk products and breakfast cereals.

Q: Why is liver so rich in vitamin A?

A: The liver is the main storage site for vitamin A in both animals and humans. So when we eat, say, chicken liver, we take in the chicken's store of vitamin A.

Q: You just referred to retinol, and I've also seen vitamin A referred to as **preformed vitamin A.** What do those terms mean?

A: Retinol and preformed vitamin A are the same thing— vitamin A in its complete form. The term preformed is used to contrast this complete form of vitamin A with **provitamin A.**

11

Q: What is provitamin A?

A: Provitamin A is a term used to describe substances in foods that the body can convert to vitamin A to satisfy its needs. In other words, these substances are precursors of vitamin A. They are also called **carotenoids**.

Q: I've heard of **beta carotene**. Is that one of the forms of provitamin A you're describing?

A: Yes. Beta carotene is a yellow-orange substance that gives color to many fruits and vegetables. Carrots, pumpkin and sweet potatoes are among the vegetables that are richest in beta carotene. Among the many fruits containing beta carotene, peaches, apricots and plums are especially rich sources. Beta carotene is also abundant in leafy green vegetables, especially kale, collard greens, spinach, chard and watercress. These foods and many others contain other carotenoids as well. Your body converts beta carotene and some other carotenoids to vitamin A as needed.

Q: I've never heard of any other carotenoids. How many are there?

A: About 600 carotenoids have been identified in fruits and vegetables, and about 60 are known to be precursors of vitamin A—substances the body can convert to vitamin A.

It's easy to get plenty of beta carotene from common vegetables. Carrots and sweet potatoes are among its richest sources. An average carrot contains about 15 milligrams of beta carotene (at about 1.5 milligrams per inch). A sweet potato contains slightly more beta carotene than a carrot in the same amount of weight—just over 2 milligrams per ounce.

Q: If there are so many carotenoids, why has beta carotene gotten so much attention?

A: Beta carotene makes up about a quarter of the carotenoid content of fruits and vegetables. So when researchers found that people eating the most fruits and vegetables had a lower risk of getting cancer and heart disease, they figured beta carotene might have something to do with it. They designed studies to determine its effectiveness, and this initial focus on beta carotene put it in the news as the researchers released their findings.

> *To optimize your carotenoid intake, choose vegetables and fruits rich in color. A dark orange carrot, for instance, contains more beta carotene than a pale one.*

Q: Did beta carotene turn out to be the reason for the health benefits of eating fruits and vegetables?

A: Results have been mixed. Many studies continue to suggest that eating foods high in beta carotene helps prevent **cardiovascular disease** and cancer. But two recent studies indicate that beta carotene **supplements** may be harmful in certain groups of people, such as smokers who also drink heavily. We explore this further in chapter 2. We also look at the results of recent research into some of the other carotenoids that abound in fruits and vegetables to see what roles they play in promoting health and preventing disease.

Q: What are some of the other common carotenoids?

A: Besides beta carotene, the carotenoids found to be most prevalent in plant foods are **lycopene, lutein** and **zeaxanthin, canthaxanthin, alpha carotene** and **cryptoxanthin.**

Q: Do all those carotenoids have beneficial effects?

A: As yet, not all have been the subjects of studies isolating their effects from those of the others. But of those that have been the subjects of such studies, among the most promising are lycopene (the dominant carotenoid in tomatoes) and lutein and zeaxanthin (which researchers often list together because they often work together; in fact, scientists were unable to isolate one from the other until recently).

Q: What does lycopene do?

A: Studies link higher blood levels of lycopene to a reduced risk of prostate, cervical, digestive tract and other cancers, as well as to a lower incidence of heart attack.

Q: How can I be sure to get lycopene?

A: Since the human body doesn't produce lycopene, we must take it in by eating lycopene-rich foods and/or taking lycopene supplements. Lycopene is found most abundantly in tomatoes, tomato products, scallions, red grapefruits, guava juice, apricots and watermelon.

Q: What about lutein and zeaxanthin?

A: The results of studies so far indicate that people who eat the most servings per week of leafy green vegetables have a lower risk of **macular degeneration**. Macular degeneration, the leading cause of blindness in people over age 65, is the age-related degeneration of a small part of the retina. Evidence linking the intake of greens to a lower incidence of this condition has opened new paths for research into a condition that otherwise has no known cause or cure.

Q: But what do greens have to do with lutein and zeaxanthin?

A: The primary carotenoids in leafy green vegetables are lutein and zeaxanthin. They are also present in the **macula** and the lens of the eye. So researchers figure that it's at least worth investigating whether these carotenoids are behind the eye protection afforded to those eating leafy greens.

Q: What foods should I eat to get lutein and zeaxanthin—just leafy greens?

A: Leafy greens are the richest sources, but significant amounts are found in other vegetables, including corn, pumpkin, celery, okra and red peppers. Eating a wide range of vegetables is your best bet.

Q: Didn't you mention some other carotenoids?

A: Yes. Canthaxanthin, a red carotenoid, is found in red, orange and yellow fruits and vegetables. Although canthaxanthin hasn't been the subject of extensive research, recent laboratory and animal studies show that it may play an important role in inhibiting the growth of cancer cells and that it can shrink skin tumors in mice. Alpha carotene and cryptoxanthin, too, are found in red, orange and yellow fruits and vegetables. Some research suggests that alpha carotene and cryptoxanthin help protect the body from cellular damage.

Q: Does it make any difference whether I get my vitamin A from retinol or its carotenoid precursors?

A: Yes, in several ways. Foods that naturally contain retinol are also high in fat, so you could boost your fat consumption too high if you ate, say, lots of egg yolks and butter. And if you were to take a high-dose retinol supplement, you might be at risk of reaching a blood level of retinol higher than the range considered healthy.

In contrast, eating fruits and vegetables gives you plenty of provitamin A (carotenoids), which your body converts to vitamin A as needed. The advice of most experts is to eat a balanced diet. Then you will get your vitamin A from a combination of animal and plant foods (unless you are a vegetarian who eats no dairy or eggs), along with many other nutrients.

> *Polar bear and seal livers are extremely rich in vitamin A because both animals eat so much fish and vitamin A is stored mostly in the liver. Arctic explorers have developed fatigue, vomiting, headache and irritability within a few hours of eating these foods!*

Q: **Is there anything I should do to help my body absorb carotenoids from the foods I eat?**

A: Recent research suggests that beta carotene and lycopene may be best absorbed when eaten with a bit of fat, such as the oil-and-vinegar dressing on a salad.

Q: **What about retinol—do I need to eat that with fat too?**

A: Yes. But the foods that naturally contain retinol originate in animals and are high in fat already. So you won't need to add extra fat to satisfy the requirement.

Q: **Why does fat help with vitamin A absorption?**

A: Vitamin A is **fat soluble**.

Q: What does that mean?

A: In order to describe how vitamins function in the body, researchers place vitamins into two groups: fat soluble and **water soluble**. It's important to know that if you consume more of a fat-soluble vitamin than your body needs, your body stores at least some of what it can't use in your liver and fatty tissues. Of the fat-soluble vitamins (A, D, E and K), vitamin A (as retinol) and vitamin D can build up to toxic levels and cause negative reactions.

Q: What kind of negative reactions?

A: Symptoms of excessive intake range from headache and flaky skin to spleen enlargement, bone thickening and joint pain. But such a high buildup is unlikely to occur in healthy people who get their preformed vitamin A from a varied diet or from both diet and moderate supplementation.

Q: What about water-soluble vitamins?

A: Water-soluble vitamins—vitamin C and the B vitamins—either are not stored in the body or are stored in small amounts. (The exception is B_{12}, which is stored in large amounts relative to its small daily requirement.) If you take in more than you can use of a water-soluble vitamin, your body gets rid of most or all of the excess in urine. This makes water-soluble vitamins unlikely to cause symptoms of **toxicity**, except at very high doses. This also means you need to take in water-soluble vitamins every day, because your body stores little or none of them (with the exception of B_{12}).

Q: Now that I know a little about the various forms of vitamin A, can you tell me something about what it does?

A: Vitamin A is essential for the normal development of eye tissue and vision in children, as well as for the formation of their bones and teeth. Our eyes use vitamin A to maintain good vision and to see in the dark. The vitamin also keeps **epithelial tissue** healthy, protecting it from the spread of bacterial infection and possibly preventing and interrupting precancerous developments in this tissue all over the body.

Q: What's epithelial tissue?

A: It's a kind of tissue that covers surfaces and lines tubes and cavities in our bodies. It serves many functions, including enclosing and protecting, producing secretions and excretions and taking in nourishment. It is found in many parts of the body, including the eyes, the skin, the cervix, the mucous membranes, and the linings of the lungs, urinary tract and gastrointestinal tract.

Q: You said vitamin A might interrupt precancerous developments. Are you saying that vitamin A can cure cancer?

A: As we discuss further in chapter 2, it does appear that **retinoids** can help the body fight some cancers. They may help prevent the recurrence of some cancers as well. As for carotenoids, many studies connect high blood levels of some carotenoids with lower rates of cancer. But whether it's accurate to claim that these carotenoids or retinoids directly prevent or cure cancer is another story.

Q: What are retinoids?

A: Retinoids are a group of about 4,000 substances related to retinol. Our bodies create some for use in cell development and **immune system** activities, among other things. Others are produced in laboratories and are called **synthetic retinoids**.

Q: Aren't there more things scientists are sure that vitamin A can do?

A: Certainly, though the degree of certainty varies. The knowledge gained from research is always growing, altering previous assertions. Much of the early research into vitamin A focused on its role in sustaining eyesight, because severe vitamin A deficiency has long been linked to eye disease and even blindness. Scientists began to suspect that vitamin A might influence the immune system as well when people in developing countries given vitamin A to prevent eye problems were found to be less likely to die from infectious disease and when they noticed other indications that vitamin A strengthens the body's ability to fight infection. They were right, though the immune-boosting effects of vitamin A are selective. Research continues to uncover how and when it works and how its capacities might translate into disease prevention or cure.

Q: Vitamin A is used to treat some skin problems, isn't it?

A: Yes. The skin often responds positively to medicinal uses of retinol. Retinol-derived prescription drugs such as isotretinoin (Accutane) can help clear up severe acne. Another retinol-derived product, tretinoin (Retin-A), can help repair sun-damaged skin. And research is under way to find whether retinoids can help treat skin cancer; some results have been promising so far, as we see in chapter 2.

Q: Does vitamin A intake have any relationship to cardiovascular disease?

A: Probably, though not as retinol but through its carotenoid precursors and other carotenoids. Numerous **population studies** indicate that a diet rich in fruits and vegetables helps lower harmful **cholesterol** levels, prevent cardiovascular disease and reduce the incidence of **stroke.** Since fruits and vegetables contain many carotenoids and some of these carotenoids are known to be **antioxidants,** scientists have reasoned that the antioxidant powers of carotenoids may best explain the heart-protective effects of fruits and vegetables.

Q: Wait a minute. What is an antioxidant?

A: An antioxidant is a substance that slows or stops oxidative reactions, or **oxidation.**

Q: And what is oxidation?

A: Oxidation is a chemical process in which a molecule combines with oxygen and loses electrons.

Q: What does losing electrons have to do with antioxidants?

A: Antioxidants help prevent and reverse undesirable oxidation in the body's cells. If you've ever studied chemistry, you may remember that atoms contain a nucleus of protons and neutrons and that this nucleus is surrounded by electrons. These electrons are negatively charged and move in pairs, which helps keep them stable. Atoms with pairs of electrons stay whole and perform their usual tasks in the body. But sometimes oxidation causes an atom or a molecule to lose one or more electrons, leading to the presence of unpaired electrons. These atoms and molecules with unpaired electrons are known as **free radicals**.

Q: What's so radical about an atom with an unpaired electron?

A: An unpaired electron upsets the balance in a molecule. So the free radical attempts to steal electrons from other molecules to regain balance. By doing this, it sets off a chain reaction, creating one free radical after another and thus breaking down many molecules.

Q: And why is that bad—what do free radicals do in the body?

A: They can destroy enzymes used to convey information throughout the body. They can destroy protein molecules and can interfere with a cell's ability to take in nutrients and expel waste, which it must do to survive. They can also damage a cell's genetic material, or DNA, so that when a cell reproduces, it creates mutations that may lead to cancer. And they can harm fat compounds in the body, causing them to turn rancid and release more free radicals. This process, called **lipid peroxidation**, is thought to be linked to the development of cardiovascular disease. Free radicals have also been connected to the deterioration that occurs as we age. As you can see, free radicals are believed to play many destructive roles.

Q: You said that free radicals are created when molecules combine with oxygen. When and why do these oxidative reactions occur?

A: Oxidative reactions take place in our bodies around the clock. Our cells use oxygen for many activities, from generating energy to manufacturing enzymes. The same cellular activities that keep us alive require oxidation and thus lead to the production of free radicals. Cells in our immune

system deliberately make free radicals for use as weapons to disable harmful invaders such as bacteria and viruses. Harmful substances in our environment, such as cigarette smoke, air pollutants and ultraviolet light, also cause oxidative reactions, leading our bodies to produce free radicals.

Q: So what does vitamin A have to do with this?

A: As retinol, probably nothing. But some of the carotenoids are known antioxidants, which means that they slow or stop oxidative reactions. Antioxidants do this by offering electrons to free radicals, stopping the free-radical chain reaction. Instead of becoming harmful themselves, antioxidants that have given up electrons become inactive.

Q: Besides carotenoids, what other antioxidants are there?

A: Other known antioxidants include vitamin E, vitamin C and the **mineral** selenium.

Q: That's the first mineral you've mentioned. What's the difference between a vitamin and a mineral?

A: Vitamins and minerals are naturally occurring nutrients in the foods we eat. **Essential vitamins** and **essential minerals** are those we must get through diet because our bodies either can't create them or can create them only in small amounts. Through research that started at the beginning of the twentieth century, about 13 essential vitamins and 15 essential minerals have been isolated in foods, as have many other substances and compounds. If you are deficient in just one of these essential vitamins or minerals, your body can't function normally. Vitamins and minerals play vital roles in just about every bodily process, including **immune response**, digestion, reproduction and mental alertness. That's why they're called essential—adequate intake is essential for human life.

Now here's the difference between them. Vitamins are organic compounds, which means they contain carbon and come from plants and animals or from substances made of living materials, such as petroleum products and coal. Minerals, in contrast, are inorganic compounds, which don't originate in organisms that were alive and don't contain carbon.

Q: So we get essential minerals and vitamins by eating plants and animals?

A: Right. We get them through a cycle of transmission. Plants derive minerals from soil and water. When we eat plants, we take in the minerals they have gleaned, as well as the vitamins that plants produce as they grow. When we eat animals and animal products such as milk, we take in the animals' stores of vitamins and minerals, gained mostly from eating plants and drinking water. For humans, too, water is a rich source of minerals. We may get some of our vitamins and minerals from supplements as well.

Q: How much vitamin A do people require?

A: Our need for this vitamin depends in part on body weight, so the recommended amounts reflect the approximate weight difference between men and women. The **Recommended Dietary Allowance (RDA)**, which is the amount considered adequate to meet the known nutrient needs of most healthy people, is 800 **RE** for women and 1,000 RE for men.

Q: What does RE stand for?

A: RE stands for **retinol equivalent**. You may remember that preformed vitamin A is called retinol and that provitamin A is converted to retinol as needed. The retinol equivalent was created so that we can talk about the amount of retinol provided, whether by preformed vitamin A or by beta carotene (the carotenoid commonly used in vitamin supplements along with or instead of retinol).

Q: But my vitamin bottle lists **I.U.** What is an **I.U.?**

A: I.U. stands for **international unit**, a unit of measure that researchers use for both vitamin A and vitamin E. Like the RE, the I.U. can be used to talk about both retinol and carotenoids.

Q: So if the RDAs of vitamin A are 800 RE for women and 1,000 RE for men, what would those amounts be in I.U.?

A: For retinol, 800 RE is equivalent to 4,000 I.U., and 1,000 RE is equivalent to 5,000 I.U. For beta carotene, 800 RE is equivalent to 8,000 I.U., and 1,000 RE is equivalent to 10,000 I.U.

Q: So do women and men need to strive for a daily intake of 800 and 1,000 RE, respectively, of vitamin A, whether in its retinol or carotenoid form?

A: Not exactly. As we said, retinol is fat soluble. That means excess is stored in your liver and fatty tissues, so you can ingest more on one day and less on the next. However, daily intake of fruits and vegetables—the sources of carotenoids—has repeatedly been shown to be crucial to optimal health.

Q: How does a person know if she's not getting enough vitamin A?

A: The first sign of a vitamin A deficiency is usually an inability of the eyes to adapt to darkness, or **night blindness**. (Eye symptoms worsen with continued deficiency, and severe deprivation can cause permanent blindness.) Other symptoms include reduced secretions of mucus, resulting in a dry mouth and other dry areas; loss of appetite; and reduced resistance to infection. In children, a deficiency can lead to stunted growth, improper bone formation and crooked teeth.

Q: Do most people get enough vitamin A?

A: It depends on which people you're talking about. In developing countries, vitamin A deficiency is very common and is linked to many symptoms of ill health, including those listed above, as well as to death from infectious diseases. In industrialized countries, people with deficiencies are likely to have less severe symptoms, such as night blindness. According to surveys of people's diets, most Americans get adequate amounts of vitamin A, although they get most of it as retinol, not as carotenoids. Carotenoids perform vital roles apart from their vitamin A activity, such as inhibiting oxidation, so increasing consumption of fruits and vegetables is widely recommended.

That said, even among generally well nourished people, some people are at higher risk of vitamin A deficiency, including alcoholics, the critically ill and the institutionalized elderly. These groups may be at higher risk because they need higher amounts, because they are unlikely to be getting adequate amounts through diet or for both reasons. People with diseases that inhibit the fat-absorbing ability of the intestines (and thus hinder absorption of fat-soluble vitamins) are also at greater risk of deficiency. These diseases include **celiac disease** and **cystic fibrosis**. Intestinal or pancreatic surgery can also impede fat absorption and the absorption of fat-soluble vitamins, including vitamin A.

Q: Is it easy to get the RDA of vitamin A from foods, whether as carotenoids or as retinol?

A: Yes, if you eat a varied, balanced diet. As far as carotenoids are concerned, if you eat the recommended three to five servings of vegetables and two to four servings of fruits per day, it would be hard not to meet or even to exceed the RDA. The average carrot contains about 5,000 I.U. of beta carotene, and a single sweet potato contains about 10,000 I.U. Yet studies suggest that very few Americans actually consume that many servings of fruits and vegetables. Instead, Americans get most of their vitamin A as retinol by eating animal foods, including meats, fish, fortified dairy products and fortified breakfast cereals.

Q: **What form of vitamin A am I likely to get when I take a multivitamin supplement?**

A: Until the early 1990s, the answer would have been retinol (preformed vitamin A). But after research into the vitamin A intake of pregnant women indicated that a high intake of retinol may raise the incidence of birth defects, manufacturers began substituting beta carotene for at least part of the retinol content of their vitamins. Because beta carotene is converted to retinol only as needed, it is considered a safer way to add to the amount of vitamin A taken in through diet, if one wishes to do so.

Q: **My multivitamin contains more than the amounts you list. Is that typical?**

A: Yes. While some multivitamin supplements provide only the RDA, many multivitamin and individual supplements contain a lot more.

Q: **Why is that?**

A: The RDAs are designed to meet the known nutrient needs of most healthy people, as we noted earlier. The goal of RDAs is to keep us from getting the symptoms of a deficiency of each nutrient. Yet many studies indicate that amounts above the RDAs of some nutrients may boost health.

Q: Do all studies show this benefit?

A: No. Some suggest that a high intake of some nutrients may make some people more likely to develop certain conditions. We look at how this relates to vitamin A in chapter 2.

Q: That's worrisome. But obviously, we need at least some amount of each essential vitamin and mineral, and it sounds like the RDAs are a little out of date. How can I find out what amounts of vitamin A and other nutrients I should take?

A: A lot of people share your curiosity, and many researchers are conducting studies aimed at finding out what the most beneficial doses of nutrients are. The National Academy of Sciences' Food and Nutrition Board is likely to take this research into account as it reviews and updates the RDAs and creates what it calls **Dietary Reference Intakes**, or **DRIs**.

Q: So the RDAs are being changed?

A: That's right. A shift in thinking has occurred as a result of research findings. The earlier notion that we needed these nutrients merely to prevent deficiency has given way to the idea that optimal intake levels may help slow aging and enhance health. This shift has reached the Food and Nutrition Board, the group that sets the RDAs.

Q: So this group is going to propose new recommended amounts?

A: Yes. It is currently reevaluating nutritional research to review and update the RDAs. The first of the new DRIs came out in August 1997. These guidelines will be introduced sporadically from now through the year 2000. The DRIs offer several types of intake recommendations for each nutrient, including revised RDAs designed not only to prevent deficiency diseases but also to decrease the risk of chronic diseases such as cancer, heart disease and osteoporosis.

The new RDAs are based in part on the Estimated Average Requirement, an amount that meets the estimated nutrient need of half the individuals in a specific group. When not enough information is available to estimate an average requirement, the DRIs establish an Adequate Intake, an amount that appears to sustain a desired indicator of health, such as an adequate level of calcium retention in bone, which is believed to prevent osteoporosis. The DRIs also include a Tolerable Upper Intake Level, the maximum amount unlikely to cause side effects in most healthy people.

Q: **Will the new DRIs recommend a higher intake of vitamin A than the current RDAs?**

A: It depends what the Food and Nutrition Board decides after looking over all the research. Given the ambivalent results of research into the effects of supplementation with retinol and beta carotene, the board may have a challenging time arriving at recommendations for vitamin A intake.

Q: **Are there any side effects from taking high doses of beta carotene or retinol?**

A: Yes. Taking high amounts of beta carotene, either in food or in supplements, may turn your skin yellow. Experts consider this a harmless side effect, and it disappears soon after very high consumption stops. The general consensus is that there's no danger of a toxic reaction to excessive beta carotene intake. However, studies of many thousands of people taking beta carotene supplements for years suggest that beta carotene supplementation may not always be beneficial to all people. We explore this further in chapter 2.

Q: What about side effects from high doses of retinol?

A: For retinol, it's important to note that tolerance levels vary for both amounts and periods of intake. In general, caution is required when taking large doses of retinol. Amounts taken in prescription pills that are meant to help clear up severe acne, for instance, can cause side effects and even toxicity, making acne drugs derived from vitamin A unsafe for long-term use in many cases. For women of child-bearing age, these pills should be taken only under a doctor's close supervision.

As for what levels cause toxicity, taking just one huge dose of vitamin A (usually defined as 250,000 I.U.) or taking large amounts (usually 50,000 I.U.) daily over time can lead to a toxic overload of retinol in the body. Again, amounts causing negative reactions vary; some people react negatively to a single dose of retinol as low as 20,000 I.U.

Q: What would happen if someone took in too much retinol regularly?

A: After excessive intake for a period of months, early symptoms of toxicity might include loss of appetite; dry, rough skin; cracked lips; and sparse, coarse hair. Joint pain is another common reaction, especially in children. Symptoms could also include amenorrhea (lack of menstrual periods), weakness, severe headache, fatigue, nausea and blurred vision. Symptoms usually disappear within about four weeks of halting excessive intake.

Q: Didn't you mention something earlier about pregnant women and retinol?

A: Yes. In fact, several groups of people should be cautious about retinol intake. Take heed of the following special cases:

- In a study of pregnant women's retinol intake, a few birth defects may have been linked to a daily intake of

40,000 I.U. or more of retinol (preformed vitamin A). As noted earlier, retinol was the type of vitamin A used in most supplements until this finding was released. In response, supplement manufacturers began using beta carotene in place of some or all of the retinol in their products. Since researchers aren't yet certain whether somewhat lower doses might also have negative effects, they recommend that women avoid taking in a lot more than the RDA of retinol if they are pregnant or are at any risk of becoming pregnant. (See chapter 3 for the RDA for pregnant women.)

• Birth control pills, or oral contraceptives, may raise blood levels of retinol. If you are on the Pill, you may want to monitor how much retinol you take in through animal foods and fortified products such as breakfast cereals.

• If you have chronic kidney failure and are undergoing dialysis, excessive retinol intake may put you at increased risk of developing bone disease. High retinol intake has been associated with the increased breakdown of bone and high levels of calcium in the blood of some people in these circumstances. Be sure to check with your doctor if you have chronic kidney failure and wish to take a retinol supplement.

• Special cautions about vitamin A intake also apply to those with liver disease and others, so it's wise to check with your doctor before taking more than the recommended amount of retinol in a supplement or using any vitamin A-derived medication, such as isotretinoin (Accutane).

Q: I've learned so much, but I still don't know a lot about recent research findings. How does vitamin A in its many forms help prevent and treat disease?

A: For the many answers to this question, we need to turn to chapter 2, where we explore research indicating the potential benefits and risks of vitamin A and the carotenoids.

2 VITAMIN A AND CAROTENOIDS AND THEIR USES

Q: You said in chapter 1 that vitamin A and the carotenoids provide health benefits. What are some of those benefits?

A: Among the many possibilities suggested by research, there is strong evidence that vitamin A and/or certain carotenoids are able to do the following:

- boost immune system function

- help protect against the initiation, growth and recurrence of cancer

- slow a process that leads to clogged arteries and heart attack

- protect the lungs against damage from smoking and cystic fibrosis

- maintain the health of the eyes, even into old age

- improve severe acne and skin damage

In addition, eating an adequate amount of fruits and vegetables, which contain many carotenoids, seems to help prevent cardiovascular disease, cancer and other diseases.

Q: That's quite a list. How strong is the evidence?

A: The strength of evidence varies from one benefit to another, and new studies continue to alter and refine the picture. But some of the above claims are based on **clinical trials**, in which vitamin A or beta carotene was used to treat people who have a particular condition. These findings are considered more definitive than, say, the results of studies based on dietary questionnaires.

Q: Why are studies based on dietary questionnaires considered less certain?

A: Studies based on dietary questionnaires don't actually pinpoint cause and effect. They simply show links that need to be further researched. A dietary study, for example, can show that people who eat lots of fruits and vegetables have a lower risk of getting cancer, but it cannot prove that a certain nutrient in fruits and vegetables actually reduces cancer risk.

In addition, some dietary surveys rely on participants' generalizations about their past intake of certain foods. If you've ever tried to remember everything you ate even just yesterday and to estimate amounts, you can imagine the risk of errors in the surveys that rely on participants' memories. To improve the reliability of studies based on food intake questionnaires, some researchers now ask participants daily for intake information.

Q: Do researchers refine their methods for other kinds of studies as well?

A: Absolutely. One reason is that research findings often conflict. Great excitement may be generated by early studies showing a positive effect, but if the studies that follow don't confirm this effect, researchers seek to understand why the results have differed. So they pay close attention to methods, not only to evaluate the reliability of studies but also

to guide their design of further studies. The lesson in all this
for us is that in most cases, we should view findings of the
health benefits of vitamin A and carotenoids as pieces of an
incomplete puzzle.

Q: Is there a chance that vitamin A and carotenoids
can do some of what you've listed earlier?

A: Definitely. And they may do more. As we said,
carotenoids seem to play a role in reducing the risk
of death from the major killers in the United States—cancer
and heart disease. Certain carotenoids seem to help prevent
these conditions, and vitamin A may help reverse some
precancerous conditions.

Q: Before we get into the details, can you remind
me what carotenoids are?

A: Sure. Carotenoids are naturally occurring, colorful
compounds that are abundant in plants; some of
these compounds can be converted to vitamin A. About 600
carotenoids have been identified, but only a small number are
found in appreciable quantities in human blood and tissues
and in the foods we eat. Of these, beta carotene, cryptoxanthin,
canthaxanthin, lycopene, and lutein and zeaxanthin are among
those known to function as antioxidants, which, you recall,
slow or stop potentially harmful oxidative reactions.

Q: Do these carotenoids need to be converted to
vitamin A before they can act as antioxidants?

A: Apparently not. Beta carotene and cryptoxanthin are
precursors of vitamin A, but canthaxanthin and lutein
are not; nevertheless, all are antioxidants. And a Japanese study
reported in a 1996 issue of *Nutrition and Cancer* indicates
that beta carotene can act as an antioxidant without being
converted to vitamin A.

Q: Is vitamin A an antioxidant too?

A: Not really, although you may read that it is. Many sources don't distinguish between vitamin A and its carotenoid precursors. When a general source refers to vitamin A as an antioxidant, it really refers to the vitamin's carotenoid precursors.

Q: How can vitamin A fight cancer if it's not an antioxidant?

A: It does so at least partly through its effects on cell multiplication and maturation. Studies to date indicate that vitamin A can help limit and even prevent cancers in some parts of the body.

Q: That's interesting. Is it the antioxidant activity of some carotenoids that helps them contribute to disease prevention?

A: Probably. Researchers are pursuing the hypothesis that antioxidants help fight disease. Their interest in carotenoids began with the many studies that link a higher intake of foods rich in carotenoids—and higher blood levels of carotenoids—to a lower risk of heart disease and cancer.

Q: Why do researchers look at both intake and blood levels? Doesn't a low intake always lead to a low blood level, and a high intake to a high level?

A: Although intake usually correlates to blood level and researchers often measure levels of nutrients in the blood to measure the effects of intake, blood levels of vitamin A, carotenoids and other nutrients are also affected by factors other than intake. For example, many diseases that affect the intestines' ability to absorb fats also affect the absorption of fat-soluble vitamins, including vitamin A. Gender, age, smoking habits and alcohol consumption can also influence blood levels of nutrients. We look further into some of these factors in chapter 3.

Q: Do researchers ever check levels of nutrients elsewhere in the body?

A: Yes. Some check tissue levels, which are considered a better indicator of long-term intake since they don't fluctuate as rapidly as blood concentrations of nutrients.

Q: Getting back to those studies of dietary intake and blood levels of carotenoids—has further research confirmed the protective benefits of carotenoids?

A: Yes and no. Studies of dietary intake continue to link a high intake of fruits and vegetables—and, consequently, a high intake of carotenoids—to lower rates of heart disease and cancer. And numerous studies indicate that people with low blood levels of carotenoids are at higher risk of heart disease and cancer than people with higher levels. But studies in which researchers have attempted to substitute supplements of beta carotene for fruits and vegetables have usually produced less promising results. Further studies suggest that other carotenoids, singly or in combination, may prove more effective at disease prevention.

Q: If that's the case, why has research focused on beta carotene?

A: There are several reasons. Because beta carotene makes up a fourth of edible carotenoids, scientists had good reason to believe it could be the source of the health benefits of fruits and vegetables. In addition, beta carotene supplements are relatively inexpensive and nontoxic, so the prospect of these supplements lowering the risk of cancer and heart disease was quite appealing. And research into other carotenoids has been difficult because information on the amounts of some other carotenoids in foods was not available until recently.

Q: Has this new information on beta carotene and other carotenoids changed the direction of research?

A: Yes. More researchers are exploring the activities of carotenoids other than beta carotene, both in the laboratory and in humans. And some studies focusing on dietary intake and blood levels of the other major carotenoids have had promising results.

VITAMIN A AND CAROTENOIDS AND THE IMMUNE SYSTEM

Q: You said vitamin A plays a role in improving immune response. Does that mean it helps keep us from getting sick?

A: Yes. The immune system defends our bodies against bacteria, viruses and other harmful invaders that cause many diseases, from infections to cancer. So a stronger response usually means less illness.

Q: What parts of the body comprise the immune system, and what do these parts do?

A: Some parts of the body produce immune system fighters, and other parts circulate them. The bone marrow and the thymus gland produce white blood cells, which are the primary soldiers of the immune system. These white blood cells circulate throughout the body in the lymphatic vessels—the immune system's own circulatory system, which permeates every organ but the brain and circulates a fluid called lymph. Some white blood cells circulate in the blood, as well as through the lymphatic vessels.

Q: What do these white blood cells do?

A: They fend off unwanted substances in the body. There are many kinds of white blood cells, each playing a particular role in immune response. The primary categories are **phagocytes** and **lymphocytes**.

Phagocytes engulf foreign substances and cellular debris; they clear the body of abnormal or old cells, cellular debris and organisms that could cause disease. Lymphocytes, which are small in comparison, generally fall into one of three types: **B lymphocytes, T lymphocytes** or **natural killer cells.**

B lymphocytes, or B cells, identify potentially harmful substances and attempt to make them harmless by producing antibodies. Antibodies attach to the substances and neutralize them, much as antioxidants neutralize free radicals.

T lymphocytes, or T cells, attack and kill invaders. They also prompt B cells to produce antibodies and produce chemicals that stimulate phagocytes to attack.

Natural killer cells, slightly larger than B and T cells, are powerful killers of germs and cancer cells. They also produce chemicals that control some activities of B cells, T cells and phagocytes.

Vitamin A and Carotenoids and Immune Response

Q: That's an impressive bunch of fighters. But what does vitamin A have to do with all this?

A: Vitamin A is essential for the normal function of the immune system. Researchers are still determining exactly what role vitamin A plays in the immune system, but the vitamin appears to regulate immune functions, including cell maturation and the activities of both phagocytes and chemicals that pass signals among the cells of the immune system (*Lancet,* January 7, 1995). Consequently, if your body doesn't get enough vitamin A, it isn't able to mount as powerful an immune response. (The immune response is what the immune system does to defend our bodies from harm; when the fighters we just described go into action, they are taking part in the immune response.)

Q: Can vitamin A improve immune response?

A: Yes. Supplementation with high doses of vitamin A has been shown to increase immune response, resistance to infection and survival in undernourished children. The evidence is strong enough that the World Health Organization recommends that children ages six months and older in developing countries receive 100,000 international units of vitamin A with their immunizations (*Lancet,* July 12, 1997). Here are a few recent studies.

- A study in Bangladesh found that some infants reacted to vaccinations with stronger immune responses when they were given vitamin A in three large monthly doses of 50,000 I.U. at the time of the vaccinations (*American Journal of Clinical Nutrition,* January 1997).

- Another study found that vitamin A supplementation in undernourished children ages six months to five years reduced death rates by 23 percent. Seeking to add results for younger children to this picture, researchers studied more than 2,000 Indonesian infants from birth. Those receiving 50,000 I.U. of vitamin A on their first day of life were less likely to die during the nearly six-month study period than were those given a **placebo**, or inactive substance. The vitamin offered significant protection against infections, the leading cause of infant death for these children (*Journal of Pediatrics,* April 1996).

- Two studies of acute respiratory infection—a leading cause of death for children in developing countries— tell more. In one, researchers found that the lower the blood levels of vitamin A in children, the more severe their respiratory infections (*South African Medical Journal,* January 1997). In the other, children under age five who were undernourished or who showed signs of a vitamin A deficiency had significantly more attacks of acute respiratory infection than those with adequate vitamin A intake (*Indian Journal of Public Health*, January-March 1996).

Q: Have researchers studied the effects of vitamin A supplementation on other groups of people?

A: Yes. Hospitals commonly give supplemental vitamin A to premature infants, who often have less mature immune systems than infants born full term. This does increase the infants' blood levels of vitamin A, but to date, no definite positive effect on rates of disease and death has been found. And at the opposite end of the age spectrum, many recent studies have focused on the elderly because immune response—particularly the activity of T cells—lessens with age.

Q: What have those studies found? Is vitamin A helpful for older people?

A: Not according to two recent studies. In one, Italian researchers gave 800 I.U. of vitamin A to elderly people to see whether T cell numbers and activity would increase. Vitamin A actually reduced some types of T cells, thus weakening an aspect of immune response in this elderly group (*Journal of the American Medical Association*, March 11, 1998). And in a British study, researchers measured blood levels of vitamin A, beta carotene and other nutrients in two groups of people—one about 80 years old and the other about 27— then exposed both groups to a foreign substance to stimulate the production of white blood cells, including B and T cells. Although blood levels of vitamin A, beta carotene and other nutrients in the elderly group equaled or exceeded those of the younger study participants, their lymphocyte response to the foreign substance was still significantly below that of the younger group (*Mechanisms of Ageing and Development*, March 1997).

Q: It seems children have had better luck when it comes to vitamin A. Does beta carotene produce better results in adults?

A: Beta carotene does appear to benefit some aspects of immunity in adults. But the research to date indicates that it has significant effects only on certain aspects of immune function and only in certain groups of people, as the following studies show:

- Investigators at Tufts University conducted two studies to test whether healthy elderly people taking beta carotene would have strengthened T cell immune responses. In one study, they gave healthy elderly women 90 milligrams of beta carotene—a very high dose—daily for three weeks. In the second study, healthy elderly men took 50 milligrams of beta carotene every other day for 10 to 12 years. In both studies, the supplements raised blood levels of beta carotene but had no effect on T cell immune response (*American Journal of Clinical Nutrition,* October 1997).

- A study published in the November 1996 *American Journal of Clinical Nutrition* found that beta carotene increases the activity of natural killer cells. Elderly men who took 50 milligrams of beta carotene every other day for 10 to 12 years had higher natural killer cell activity than those who took a placebo. Middle-aged men participating in the study showed no significant boost in their natural killer cell activity.

- Beta carotene and other carotenoids may boost immune response to human papillomavirus (HPV), a common sexually transmitted virus that can lead to cervical cancer. To determine why HPV infections go away in some women and not in others, researchers measured blood levels of antioxidant nutrients, including five carotenoids, in nonsmoking women with HPV. Blood levels of beta carotene, cryptoxanthin, lutein and vitamin E were 24 percent lower in women with the most persistent HPV infections. Women with persistent infections are at higher risk of getting cervical cancer

(Cancer Epidemiology, Biomarkers and Prevention, November 1997).

Q: ● Have there been any other studies of beta carotene and immune response?

A: ● Yes. In fact, some have found that beta carotene may boost immune response in ways that might strengthen the body's defenses against cancer in particular.

- In a study conducted at the Institute of Food Research in the United Kingdom, researchers gave participants 50 milligrams of beta carotene (the equivalent of three or four carrots) daily for a month. The researchers found that beta carotene stimulated a molecule that helps the immune system target and destroy cancer cells (*Cancer Weekly,* January 6, 1997).

- A group of healthy, nonsmoking adult men were given either 15 milligrams of beta carotene or a placebo for about two months. Not only did blood levels of beta carotene increase in those taking beta carotene, but so did levels of **monocytes,** white blood cells that control some tumor-fighting aspects of immune response (*Journal of Laboratory and Clinical Medicine,* March 1997).

- In a study conducted at Loyola University Medical Center, researchers analyzed blood samples of healthy people and people who had been treated for precancer or cancer of the colon before and after giving them 30 milligrams of beta carotene daily for three months. Before supplementation, the cancer patients had less T cell activity. After supplementation, the cancer patients showed significant increases in T cell activity. Beta carotene didn't affect T cell activity in healthy people or in people with precancer of the colon, however (*Nutrition and Cancer,* 1997).

Vitamin A and Carotenoids and Cancer

Q: Those studies do show increases in some kinds of immune response for some people, but I don't understand how that relates to protection against cancer. Could you clarify the link between increased immune response and cancer?

A: Sure. The many types of cells that make up the immune system work together to target potentially cancer-causing substances and abnormal cells. By identifying and destroying these substances and cells, the immune system prevents them from leading to cancer. So boosting immune function—such as increasing T cell activity—strengthens the body's defenses against cancer.

Q: Generally speaking, what can vitamin A and the carotenoids do to combat cancer?

A: In different ways and under some circumstances, they can actually protect against the development of cancer and its recurrence, help control precancerous and cancerous conditions and boost the effectiveness of chemotherapy.

Cancer develops when cells lose their normal control mechanisms and begin to grow and multiply abnormally. The control mechanisms in cancerous cells have been damaged by carcinogens, cancer-causing agents that include chemicals, viruses, radiation and sunlight. Vitamin A and some carotenoids may be able to help the body fix or destroy these damaged cells. And some carotenoids can restore balance to free radicals, preventing these cells from causing damage that could lead to cancer.

Vitamin A and Carotenoids and Cancer Risk

Q: That's exciting. What do studies show about these anticancer powers?

A: For vitamin A, many animal studies and some human studies show that retinoids are effective at cancer prevention and suppression.

As for carotenoids, many studies link a high consumption of fruits and vegetables rich in beta carotene and/or high blood levels of carotenoids to a lower rate of cancers of the lung, bladder, breast, cervix, endometrium and rectum, as well as **melanoma**, a cancer that starts in the pigment-producing cells of the skin and can spread quickly (*Primary Care and Cancer,* February 1994). Further, a 1997 review of the results of studies of dietary intake of beta carotene, reported in *Nutrition and Cancer,* suggests that foods high in beta caro-tene—which contain a mix of carotenoids—prevent the initiation or growth of cancers.

Q: Before we go on, could you remind me what retinoids are?

A: Sure. Retinoids are a group of substances related to retinol, or vitamin A. Some can be created in our bodies; others have been produced in laboratories and are called synthetic retinoids. There are more than 4,000 retinoids, with a broad range of activities, toxicity levels, sites of effective action and other characteristics. Retinoids influence many body processes, including cell development and immune sys-tem activity. They show much potential as anticancer agents, helping some abnormal, potentially cancerous cells to become normal again.

Lung Cancer

: **What cancers have researchers looked at in relation to the preventive effects of retinoids and carotenoids?**

A: Some of the most current studies have focused on cancers of the lung, breast, colon and rectum, liver, prostate and skin. Let's look at each of these cancers separately, starting with lung cancer, since many studies have addressed the effects of retinoids, vitamin A and the carotenoids on lung cancer risk. (Throughout the book, we use the term vitamin A when we are referring to retinol or retinoids unless we're referring to a specific retinoid.) Results from supplementation have been mixed, but the benefits of eating fruits and vegetables are certain. Let's look at the positive results first.

- Investigators at Johns Hopkins University compared the blood levels of carotenoids in more than 250 people with lung cancer with those of more than 500 healthy people. They found significantly lower blood concentrations of cryptoxanthin, beta carotene, lutein and zeaxanthin among the lung cancer group, suggesting that these people ate fewer fruits and vegetables (*Cancer Epidemiology, Biomarkers and Prevention*, November 1997).

- A long-term study of nearly 2,000 middle-aged men found that those who ate the fewest foods containing beta carotene had up to a 48 percent higher risk of developing lung cancer than those who ate the most of these foods. The lowest risk of lung cancer was found in men taking in at least 5,000 I.U. (about 3 milligrams) of beta carotene daily from foods—less than the amount that supplies the RDA of vitamin A (*Medical Tribune*, August 6, 1992).

- Researchers studied dietary intake of carotenoids and vitamins E, C and A in relation to lung cancer rates using data from the First National Health and Nutrition Examination Survey Epidemiologic Follow-up Study, which involved about 4,000 men and 6,000 women. While vitamin A had no effect on lung cancer risk, carotenoids did offer protection. Those who took in the most carotenoids, vitamin E and vitamin C were 68 percent less likely to get lung cancer than those who took in the least. Among smokers, those who took in the most carotenoids were 50 percent less likely to get lung cancer. And those who smoked the least saw their risk cut by 77 percent (*American Journal of Epidemiology*, August 1, 1997).

Q: These findings about blood levels and dietary intake are encouraging. But wasn't there something in the news a few years ago about beta carotene supplements *increasing* the risk of lung cancer?

A: There have been several such reports. Two very large studies of beta carotene and/or vitamin A supplementation found higher rates of lung cancer in some groups of people who took supplements.

The most recent of these studies, the Beta-Carotene and Retinol Efficacy Trial (CARET), in which more than 18,000 men and women at high risk of developing lung cancer took either 30 milligrams of beta carotene and 25,000 I.U. of vitamin A or a placebo daily, was stopped 21 months early, after about four years of supplementation. The study was designed to find out whether the supplements would reduce lung cancer in the high-risk group tested: smokers and workers exposed to asbestos. But instead, 25 percent more lung cancers occurred among those taking the supplements compared with those taking the placebo (*New England Journal of Medicine*, May 2, 1996).

Even though beta carotene supplements didn't help many men in the CARET study, the study did confirm a finding made in many dietary studies: Those who started out with higher blood beta carotene levels had lower risks of cancer and heart disease, whether or not they took supplements in the study.

The results echo those of a widely publicized 1994 Finnish study in which male smokers taking beta carotene supplements experienced 18 percent more lung cancers than smokers taking a placebo. The study—one of the first to look at the effects of beta carotene supplements—prompted news reports that beta carotene may actually cause lung cancer. It also prompted cautions from members of the research community, who pointed out that there was more evidence of benefit than harm from beta carotene. In fact, the researchers who conducted the study speculated that the negative finding may have been due to chance (*New England Journal of Medicine*, April 14, 1994).

Q: ● **I guess chance is an unlikely cause at this point, now that a second study has found the same thing. But could you refresh my memory about that Finnish study? I do remember reading about it.**

A: ● Sure. The study, known as the Alpha-Tocopherol Beta Carotene (ATBC) Cancer Prevention Study, involved more than 29,000 Finnish male smokers, ages 50 to 69, who took 20 milligrams of beta carotene, 50 milligrams of vitamin E, both or a placebo daily for five to eight years. Those who took beta carotene, whether with vitamin E or without, had higher rates of lung, prostate and stomach cancers than those who took the placebo.

But not all the beta carotene findings in this study were negative. Men whose blood levels and dietary intake of beta carotene were highest at the start of the study—before supplementation began—had a lower rate of lung cancer than those who started the study with lower blood and intake levels, regardless of whether they took supplements. Higher baseline blood levels of beta carotene were also linked to a lower rate of cancer in the CARET study.

Q: Maybe beta carotene's negative effect is limited to certain people. Has anyone looked deeper into the link between beta carotene and the higher lung cancer rates?

A: Yes. A second report on the CARET study focused on the lung cancer increase, looking for factors that may have helped determine who got the disease. Researchers found no link between high blood levels of beta carotene and lung cancer risk, indicating that high blood levels of beta carotene were not the cause of the increase in lung cancer. But they did find that the people in the beta carotene and vitamin A group who drank the most alcohol were 99 percent more likely to get lung cancer than those taking the placebo—an enormous difference in risk and perhaps the beginning of a partial explanation of the study's negative results.

The investigators advised current smokers and asbestos-exposed workers not to take beta carotene supplements or the combination of beta carotene and vitamin A. But they also released a new piece of evidence indicating that the supplements may have helped some participants: Former smokers with no history of asbestos exposure who took beta carotene and vitamin A during the study had a 20 percent reduction in lung cancer risk (*Journal of the National Cancer Institute,* November 6, 1996).

Q: That's interesting. Have any other large studies looked at beta carotene supplements and lung cancer risk?

A: Yes. In the Physicians' Health Study, more than 22,000 male doctors took 50 milligrams of beta carotene or a placebo every other day. The group included current and former smokers, but all were healthy at the start. Beta carotene had no effect on the incidence of lung cancer and other cancers. The study lasted an average of 12 years— longer than the five- to 10-year development period for many cancers—giving beta carotene a fair chance to have an effect if it were going to do so (*New England Journal of Medicine,* May 2, 1996).

Q: So what do these three big studies say about beta carotene supplements and lung cancer risk?

A: When the results of the ATBC and CARET studies are combined, beta carotene supplements are linked to a 20 percent increase in lung cancer risk for smokers, former smokers and people exposed to asbestos. The increase drops to 16 percent when data from the Physicians' Health Study—which studied both smokers and nonsmokers—are added (*Journal of the National Cancer Institute,* November 6, 1996). True, that 16 percent increase was derived from studies in which the majority of participants were at higher risk of developing lung cancer than the general population. Nevertheless, it is a sobering statistic.

Q: If beta carotene can produce such negative results, why did researchers use it in those studies?

A: Researchers didn't expect such negative results; in fact, they had several reasons to believe that beta carotene would have a positive effect on lung cancer risk. For starters, many studies of fruit and vegetable intake showed that people who ate the most of these foods—which are rich in beta carotene—had the lowest risk of lung cancer. Because data about food levels of other carotenoids were hard to come by until recently, many of these studies attributed the benefits of fruit and vegetable intake to beta carotene. Between 1983 and 1993, more than two dozen published studies found a link between beta carotene intake and a lower risk of lung cancer. The reports indicated anywhere from a 10 to a 70 percent drop in the risk of lung cancer in people with diets high in beta carotene.

Another reason is that vitamin A and those carotenoids that can be converted to vitamin A—including beta carotene—are vital for the normal development and maintenance of the lungs and other respiratory tissues. Since healthy tissues fight disease better, it made sense to think that this role, along with their role in immune function, made vitamin A and carotenoids likely candidates for lung cancer prevention.

But to find out if beta carotene really does have a role in cancer prevention, researchers needed to conduct **chemo-**

prevention trials—studies in which people are given either a substance suspected of preventing cancer (in this case, beta carotene) or a placebo to determine if those given the test substance are less likely to come down with cancer than those given the placebo. All three of the big studies we just looked at were chemoprevention trials.

Q: Well, they certainly didn't show a protective effect. Has anyone looked at why beta carotene had such negative results in certain groups of people?

A: Yes. One explanation researchers are considering is that beta carotene acted as a **pro-oxidant**—an agent that increases oxidation, thus possibly encouraging the development of disease, including cancer.

Q: Wait a minute. I thought beta carotene is an antioxidant. How can it promote oxidation?

A: Beta carotene is an antioxidant, but under certain circumstances—circumstances researchers are still identifying—antioxidants can act as pro-oxidants. In the case of beta carotene, Italian researchers have found that it acts as an antioxidant at the pressure of oxygen in normal air, but that it can act as a pro-oxidant at about five times that pressure (*Cancer Weekly Plus,* January 6, 1997). Because smoking and other injuries to lung tissue cause increased oxidation and might change oxygen pressure, some CARET researchers speculate that the pro-oxidant capacity of beta carotene may explain the harmful effects they found (*New England Journal of Medicine,* May 2, 1996).

Q: Did the negative results from CARET and ATBC lead other researchers to stop using beta carotene in their research?

A: Yes. The news sent a general alarm through those doing similar research, including the leaders of the

Women's Health Study, who had been investigating the effects
of beta carotene, vitamin E and aspirin on the risk of heart
disease and cancer in 40,000 women. While the CARET study
included only about 6,000 women and the ATBC study and
Physicians' Health Study participants were all men, the
Women's Health Study investigators found the results strong
enough that they stopped the beta carotene part of their
study (*Harvard Women's Health Watch*, March 1996).

Q: Have any studies using beta carotene
supplements continued?

A: Yes. Results were recently released from an Australian
study in which more than 1,200 former asbestos workers took either 30 milligrams of beta carotene or 25,000 I.U. of
vitamin A daily as part of a cancer prevention program. While
beta carotene didn't have negative effects in this group, it
didn't have positive ones either. However, vitamin A did have
a positive effect. Those taking vitamin A were 76 percent less
likely to develop **mesothelioma** (a tumor in the lung area that
was the most common cause of death in the study) than those
taking beta carotene. Those taking vitamin A had a higher rate
of death from cardiovascular disease, however (*International
Journal of Cancer*, January 30, 1998).

Q: Getting back to the women's health study you
just mentioned—it just occurred to me that those
big studies we discussed earlier involved mostly
men. Has anyone looked at whether carotenoids
and vitamin A have any effects on cancers
particular to women?

A: Yes. Studies have found a link between high consumption of fruits and vegetables and/or high blood levels
of vitamin A and lowered incidence of endometrial and cervical cancers. And many studies have explored whether vitamin A and carotenoid consumption reduces breast cancer risk.

Breast Cancer

Q: Could we look at some of those breast cancer studies?

A: Sure. Some show that fruit and vegetable intake reduces the risk of breast cancer, but others find that this isn't true for all age-groups. Studies of vitamin A intake also contradict: While one shows a decrease in risk, another shows an increase, and a third shows no effect at all.

- A study published in a 1997 issue of *Nutrition and Cancer* explored the effects of dietary intake of carotenoids and vitamin A on more than 5,000 women in Italy, half of whom had breast cancer and half of whom had no history of the disease or any related condition. Raw vegetables (which are high in beta carotene and other carotenoids) were most protective for *pre*menopausal women, while fish (which are high in vitamin A) were most protective for *post*menopausal women. The researchers concluded that beta carotene was most protective in younger women and became less protective with age.

- About 12,000 women in four states in the United States filled out food questionnaires for three years. Those who reported eating carrots or spinach more than twice weekly were 44 percent less likely to get breast cancer than those reporting no intake of these two vegetables. No link was found to foods containing vitamin A (*Cancer Epidemiology, Biomarkers and Prevention,* November 1997).

- In a study of premenopausal women with and without breast cancer, researchers found that the risk of breast cancer was 54 percent lower in women who consumed the most vegetables than in women who took in the least. The risk was 54 percent lower in those with the highest intake of beta carotene, 53 percent lower in those with the highest intake of lutein and zeaxanthin and 33 percent lower in those with the highest intake of alpha carotene (*Journal of the National Cancer Institute,* March 20, 1996).

- In the Netherlands Cohort Study, intake of beta carotene, vitamin A, vegetables, fruits, other foods and vitamins was examined in more than 62,000 post-menopausal women over a four-year period. Researchers found that the incidence of breast cancer was not influenced by the intake of beta carotene or of vegetables in general. Fruit consumption had a modest risk-reducing effect. For vitamin A, high intake actually led to a modest increase in breast cancer incidence (*British Journal of Cancer,* 1997).

- In an animal study, rats were given either a tomato extract rich in lycopene or supplemental beta carotene before and after they were treated with a chemical that induces breast tumors. Those rats given the tomato extract developed significantly fewer and smaller tumors than unsupplemented rats; beta carotene had no protective effect (*Cancer Detection and Prevention,* 1997).

Q: **Lycopene sounds like it might be promising. But how can I make sense of the contradictory evidence for beta carotene and vitamin A?**

A: The evidence isn't entirely contradictory. The four-state study finding that older women got no protection from beta carotene is actually consistent with the Italian study, which showed that beta carotene was less protective for postmenopausal women. However, the Italian study found a protective effect for fish consumption in older women, and true, this does seem to contradict the four-state study's finding that vitamin A may have slightly increased the subjects' risk of developing breast cancer. (As you may recall, fish oil contains vitamin A.)

Q: Those studies focused on intake, but you said earlier that such studies aren't necessarily definitive. **Have researchers conducted any other types of studies to determine whether vitamin A and carotenoids protect against breast cancer?**

A: Yes. Researchers have examined the relationship between breast cancer and levels of vitamin A and carotenoids in blood and breast tissue. But here again, the results have been contradictory.

- Researchers compared the blood of healthy women with that of women diagnosed with breast cancer. They found that while higher blood levels of lycopene, lutein and zeaxanthin were associated with a lower risk of cancer, higher blood levels of alpha carotene, beta carotene and vitamin A offered no protective effect (*Cancer Causes and Control,* March 1998).

- Researchers at the Harvard School of Public Health compared the concentrations of vitamin A and carotenoids in the breast tissue of 46 women with breast cancer with those of 63 women with noncancerous breast conditions. They found that higher tissue concentrations of these nutrients were linked to lower disease rates. The most protection came from vitamin A, beta carotene, lycopene, lutein and zeaxanthin. But while tissue levels of vitamin A and carotenoids were lower overall in women with breast cancer, tissue levels were only slightly related or were unrelated to intake, leading researchers to suggest that women with breast cancer may differ from others in how their bodies store or use up these nutrients (*American Journal of Clinical Nutrition,* September 1997).

- A study using food questionnaires and tissue measurements confirmed the Harvard study's finding. It, too, showed that women with higher tissue levels of carotenoids had a lower risk of getting breast cancer. (This study also reported a 50 percent lower breast cancer risk among premenopausal women who consumed the most beta carotene or lutein and zeaxanthin

compared with those who consumed the least.) Yet
in another study, scientists observed no association between total vitamin A concentration (combined vitamin A and carotenoids) in breast tissue and breast
cancer risk (*American Journal of Clinical Nutrition,*
September 1997).

As you can see, additional research on the relationship
between vitamin A and the carotenoids and breast cancer is
clearly needed.

Colorectal Cancer

Q: Are there conflicting results about the roles
of carotenoids and vitamin A for every kind
of cancer?

A: For some more than others. Beta carotene supplements
may or may not be helpful for colorectal cancer, for
instance, but fruits and vegetables do seem to offer protection.

When Italian researchers looked at the dietary habits of
nearly 2,000 people with colorectal cancer and 4,000 with no
history of cancer, they found that those who took in the most
beta carotene, riboflavin and vitamin C through diet had the
lowest rate of colorectal cancer (*International Journal of
Cancer,* November 14, 1997). And a study of people at high risk
of getting colon cancer found a 35 percent lower rate of colon
cell multiplication—a sign that cancer is likely to develop—
among those eating the most fruits and vegetables compared
with those eating the least (*Cancer Epidemiology, Biomarkers
and Prevention,* December 1997).

Q: What did the studies of beta carotene
supplementation find?

A: As we said, the results of these studies are contradictory. In the Australian Polyp Prevention Trial,
investigators compared people taking beta carotene supplements with those taking a placebo. They found fewer abnormal
cells that could lead to **polyps** (protruding growths) and can-

cer in those people who took the supplements (*Journal of the National Cancer Institute,* December 6, 1995). But in a study in which people with colon cancer, colon polyps and normal colons were given either 30 milligrams of beta carotene or a placebo daily, the supplements had no effect on the rate of cell multiplication, even though they caused a significant increase in beta carotene concentrations in both blood and colon tissues in all participants (*Journal of the National Cancer Institute,* January 18, 1995).

Q: Is there any other evidence to consider?

A: Yes. Several animal studies show a protective effect for beta carotene, while one indicates that other carotenoids are more beneficial.

- Researchers studied the effects of beta carotene and vitamin E-rich wheat germ on the development of abnormal colon cell clusters—which can lead to tumors—in rats on a high-fat diet, a diet that increases the risk of colon cancer. When the rats were exposed to a chemical that causes abnormal cell growth in the colon, beta carotene and wheat germ—both separately and together—protected against the development of abnormal cell clusters (*Carcinogenesis,* January 1995).

- Rats given beta carotene and vitamin E supplements or a placebo were exposed to a cancer-causing agent and fed a high-fat diet. The number of abnormal colon cell clusters and colon tumors was significantly lower in the rats that received the supplements (*Cancer Letters,* May 4, 1995).

- A Japanese study of the effects of carotenoids on the development of abnormal colon cell clusters in rats found that lycopene, lutein, alpha carotene and palm carotenes (the latter a mixture of alpha carotene, beta carotene and lycopene) restricted the development of abnormal cell clusters, while beta carotene did not. Small doses of lycopene and lutein proved especially effective, which the researchers say means that the nutrients may prevent cancer of the colon (*Cancer Letters,* October 1, 1996).

Liver Cancer

Q: Do carotenoids help prevent or minimize other types of cancer in animals?

A: Yes. Carotenoids in general appear to be beneficial for liver cancer, although studies of the benefits of individual carotenoids are contradictory.

- In a study of liver cancer prevention, investigators gave rats beta carotene, vitamin A or neither while treating them with a potent inducer of liver cancer. Only beta carotene restricted precancerous growths in the liver (*International Journal for Vitamin and Nutrition Research,* 1995).

- Researchers gave rats beta carotene along with an inducer of liver cancer and found that beta carotene protected the genetic material in cells from harm. Damaged genetic material is one cause of the abnormal cell growth and speedy cell multiplication that can lead to cancer (*British Journal of Cancer,* 1997).

- Conversely, a third study with rats, reported in a 1997 issue of *Nutrition and Cancer,* found no protective effect from beta carotene. Researchers found that lycopene, instead of beta carotene, decreased precancerous growths in the liver.

Prostate Cancer

Q: Has lycopene shown any cancer-protective effects for people?

A: Yes. Perhaps the most exciting recent finding comes from a study of prostate cancer risk. Researchers kept track of the diets and health of nearly 48,000 men for six years as part of the Health Professionals Follow-up Study. While intakes of beta carotene, alpha carotene, lutein and cryptoxanthin had no effect on prostate cancer risk, foods rich in lycopene had protective power. Men who ate a combined 10 servings of tomatoes, tomato sauce, tomato juice and pizza—the source of about 80 percent of the lycopene in their diets—per week had 35 percent fewer prostate cancers than those who ate one-and-a-half servings of these foods per week. The researchers cited a related study of Seventh-Day Adventists that also found a lower rate of prostate cancer in those eating the most tomatoes (*Journal of the National Cancer Institute,* December 6, 1995).

Q: Do other studies confirm a benefit from tomato products?

A: Yes. At a 1997 symposium on the subject of the cancer-preventing powers of cooked tomato products, investigators from leading U.S. and European research institutions reported benefits from tomato products. The cancers these foods appear to protect against most are prostate and digestive tract cancers (*Cancer Weekly Plus,* March 17, 1997).

Q: Is lycopene definitely responsible for the positive effects of eating tomato products?

A: No. But lycopene is the main carotenoid in tomatoes and a powerful antioxidant, more powerful than beta carotene. According to a 1997 article in the *American Journal of Clinical Nutrition,* many studies have linked lycopene to cancer-preventing effects. While studies examining dietary intake alone have found mixed results for lycopene, those measuring blood levels have linked higher blood lycopene levels to a lower cancer risk. And an article in the April 1997 *Journal of the American College of Nutrition* notes that both blood levels and intake of lycopene have been shown to have a strongly protective effect against prostate, pancreatic and some stomach cancers.

Q: Doesn't it seem likely, then, that lycopene is the cause of the positive effects of tomato products?

A: Yes. But you'll remember it also seemed likely that beta carotene was the cause of the positive effects of eating fruits and vegetables before studies indicated that other carotenoids and other nutrients altogether might be just as important, if not more so. As the authors of the Health Professionals Follow-up Study report remind us, the positive effects of tomato products may come from "other compounds in tomatoes, many yet to be characterized."

Q: Does vitamin A have any effect on prostate cancer risk?

A: Actually, several studies have found that high dietary vitamin A intake *increases* the incidence of prostate cancer, especially in men who are age 70 or older. In the Health Professionals Follow-up Study, men 70 or older who ate the most vitamin A-rich foods, particularly liver and cold breakfast cereals, had a higher likelihood of getting prostate cancer, while younger men were unaffected by dietary vitamin A intake. Because the results were hard to interpret—supplements of vitamin A and some vitamin A-rich foods, such as milk and eggs, had no negative effects—the researchers did not caution older men against eating vitamin A-rich foods.

Skin Cancer

Q: Didn't you say that vitamin A may help prevent skin cancer?

A: We did. One recent study indicates that vitamin A can lower the incidence of **squamous cell carcinoma**— a type of skin cancer that starts in the middle layer of the **epidermis**—although another study found no effect.

The first study mentioned above, the Southwest Skin Cancer Prevention Study, involved 2,300 people who had already had skin cancer or precancer. Participants took either 25,000 I.U. of vitamin A or a placebo daily for up to five years, and researchers tracked their health for another four years. Those who took vitamin A had 25 percent fewer new squamous cell carcinomas. But vitamin A did not affect the incidence of **basal cell carcinoma**, a type of cancer that starts in the lowest layer of the epidermis (*Cancer Epidemiology, Biomarkers and Prevention,* November 1997).

In the other, smaller study, people with histories of at least four skin cancers took 25,000 I.U. of vitamin A, 5 to 10 milligrams of the retinoid isotretinoin (Accutane, a drug used to treat severe acne) or a placebo daily for three years. No differences appeared among the three groups in terms of the length of their cancer-free period or the total number of tumors (*Cancer Epidemiology, Biomarkers and Prevention,* November 1997).

Q: Do carotenoids help prevent skin cancer?

A: According to a 1992 report in *Nutrition and Cancer,* a high intake of foods rich in both carotenoids and vitamin A, including vegetables and fish, leads to a significantly lower risk of skin cancer. In at least one study, those people who got skin cancer had lower blood levels of beta carotene and vitamin A than those who did not, suggesting that these nutrients offer protection against skin cancer.

Vitamin A and Carotenoids and Cancer Treatment

Q: We've looked at whether vitamin A and the carotenoids can help reduce cancer risk. Could we now examine some of the ways vitamin A and carotenoids have been used to treat cancer?

A: Good idea. Let's start with vitamin A and epithelial tissue, which lines tubes and cavities and covers surfaces on the inside and outside of the body, including the mouth, the cervix, the skin and parts of the lungs and respiratory system. The tissue needs vitamin A to function properly and to fight infection and other threats. When vitamin A has been used in animal studies to treat cancerous epithelial tissue, it has actually slowed or even reversed the progression of cancer (*Cancer Research,* January 1, 1998).

In humans, vitamin A has helped treat cancerous and precancerous growths in epithelial tissue in the mouth and the cervix (*Drug Therapy,* July 1992). Vitamin A can also help in the treatment of melanoma by slowing its growth. And researchers are developing retinoid creams for reversing precancerous and cancerous growths in epithelial tissue (*Drugs,* March 1997).

Q: **It sounds like vitamin A has a lot to offer epithelial tissue. What does it do for the mouth?**

A: It can help protect smokers against **oral leukoplakia,** a condition characterized by precancerous white lesions in the mouth. In a study comparing the effects of beta carotene supplementation with the effects of a low dose of the retinoid isotretinoin (Accutane) on the lesions of people with advanced oral leukoplakia, 55 percent of those taking beta carotene saw their conditions worsen compared with only 8 percent of those taking isotretinoin (*Journal of the National Cancer Institute,* February 5, 1997).

Q: **Has vitamin A been used to treat cancers elsewhere in the body besides epithelial tissue?**

A: Yes. Investigators have reported some very encouraging results for liver and lung cancers, as well as for **promyelocytic leukemia,** a life-threatening disease in which immune system cells stop developing correctly and become cancerous.

- Japanese researchers successfully used a synthetic retinoid called polyprenoic acid with liver cancer patients. Equal numbers were given polyprenoic acid or a placebo. After three years, those who took the retinoid had developed only seven tumors, while those who took the placebo had developed 20 (Associated Press, June 12, 1996).

- Patients treated with 300,000 I.U. of vitamin A daily for a year after surgery for lung cancer developed 11 percent fewer lung tumors and had one-tenth as many tumors in new locations compared with patients who received a placebo (*Journal of Clinical Oncology*, July 1993).

- In the latest study on promyelocytic leukemia, doctors compared the effectiveness of treatment with the retinoid all-trans-retinoic acid against conventional chemotherapy. Sixteen percent more of the patients who received the retinoid experienced complete remission, and overall, more people given the retinoid survived (*Internal Medicine News*, February 1, 1998).

In the next several years, we should know the results of other studies examining vitamin A's cancer-treating abilities, including worldwide trials using vitamin A as a treatment for breast cancer.

Q: Didn't you say that vitamin A has also been used with chemotherapy?

A: Yes. In the early 1980s, some studies of women with breast cancer found that chemotherapy was more effective in women with higher blood levels of vitamin A and carotenoids. Perhaps partly because of these and similar studies, vitamin A is sometimes used in combination with chemotherapy to treat breast cancer and colon cancer.

Q: Does beta carotene show any promise in treating cancer?

A: Yes. Like vitamin A, beta carotene appears to help reduce cancerous growths on the cervix (*Drug Therapy*, July 1992). And a study using 30 milligrams of beta carotene a day as a postsurgery treatment for people with colon cancer found that the colon cell multiplication rate dropped by nearly half after a month and by more than half after nine weeks. (As we mentioned earlier, a high rate of cell multiplication in the colon is a risk factor for colon cancer.) The lower rate of cell multiplication continued for six months after supplementation stopped (*Cancer Research,* August 15, 1993).

Another study, reported in a 1995 issue of *Nutrition and Cancer,* found that people with colon cancer had lower tissue stores of beta carotene than did healthy people or people with colon polyps; supplementation with 30 milligrams of beta carotene a day raised their tissue levels. Because increased tissue levels of beta carotene may improve the health of tissues, this finding suggests that beta carotene supplementation is a possible treatment for colon cancer.

Cancer-Fighting Mechanisms of Vitamin A and Carotenoids

Q: So exactly how does vitamin A help prevent or treat cancer?

A: Vitamin A's anticancer effects appear to result in part from its ability to correct the maturation and multiplication processes of precancerous and cancerous cells. Researchers have seen these effects both in test tubes and in people. Also, vitamin A can lead immune system cells to begin the process of breaking down and destroying precancerous and cancerous cells, which can limit the growth of tumors (*FASEB Journal,* July 1996).

Q: If vitamin A can correct such cellular problems, does that mean the problems themselves are related to a deficiency of vitamin A?

A: Possibly, but not always. Faulty cell formation may sometimes result from cells becoming unable to make use of vitamin A. In a test-tube study at Cornell University, human skin cancer cells had a much lower ability than normal cells to convert vitamin A into the forms needed for regulating cell growth and maturation. It is possible that this inability could be the cause of the abnormal cell growth that led the cells to become cancerous (*Cancer Research,* January 1, 1998).

Q: Do researchers have any ideas about how carotenoids might help prevent or treat cancer?

A: Yes. One theory is that the antioxidant activity of carotenoids protects us against many diseases, including cancer. And evidence does show that this can be so. But as we have seen, antioxidants can act as pro-oxidants as well, and research thus far hasn't led to a clear picture of when, why and how this switch occurs (*Lancet,* January 7, 1995).

Another theory is that carotenoids may strengthen aspects of the immune response. Many studies of animals and of human cells in laboratories suggest that beta carotene can boost T cell immune response, but results in humans haven't always confirmed this. In fact, those two big studies with negative results, ATBC and CARET, suggest that beta carotene supplements may lower T cell immune response in high-risk groups. Both lung cancer and cardiovascular disease are likely to be kept in check by T cell immune response (*American Journal of Clinical Nutrition,* October 1997).

Q: Are there any more specific ideas about how carotenoids achieve their cancer-protective effects?

A: Yes. The studies that follow suggest that some carotenoids may prevent genetic damage to cells, reduce the activity of enzymes that activate potentially cancer-causing substances and cells and promote tumors, and more.

- German researchers gave people tomato juice (in which lycopene is the dominant carotenoid), carrot juice (which is richest in alpha and beta carotene) and dried spinach powder (in which lutein and zeaxanthin dominate) separately for two weeks. Each food significantly decreased naturally occurring genetic damage to lymphocytes. Carrot juice also significantly reduced oxidation-related damage to genetic material in cells (*Carcinogenesis,* September 1997).

- Research from the University of Hawaii suggests that lutein reduces the activity of a liver enzyme responsible for activating carcinogens (*Pharmacogenetics*, February 1997).

- Supplements of beta carotene (20 milligrams per day) decreased the activity of an enzyme that promotes tumors in the gastrointestinal tract by 50 percent in people at increased risk of stomach cancer (*Cancer, Epidemiology Biomarkers Preview*, December 1995).

- For two weeks, Japanese researchers gave canthaxanthin or beta carotene to mice with skin cancer. The skin tumors shrank, and the levels of an altered gene that can make normal cells turn cancerous dropped in these tumors (*Nutrition and Cancer*, 1996).

- A test-tube study conducted in Italy found that canthaxanthin restricted cell multiplication in colon cancer and melanoma cells taken from humans. The researchers also discovered that canthaxanthin prompted a process, **apoptosis**, that helps limit the growth of tumors by breaking down and destroying cells (*Carcinogenesis*, February 1998). You may remember that we said vitamin A has this capacity as well. This ability may explain why vitamin A and some carotenoids can increase the effectiveness of chemotherapy—another process aimed at breaking down and destroying tumor cells (*Nutrition and Cancer*, 1997).

Q: Could you help me put all this in perspective by reminding me what positive effects vitamin A has so far been found to have on cancer?

A: Certainly. Forms of vitamin A have reversed some precancerous lesions (including oral leukoplakia), reduced the size and number of some tumors and suppressed the recurrence of cancer. Various studies have suggested that forms of vitamin A may even block the development of cancer in epithelial tissue (*Cancer Epidemiology, Biomarkers and Prevention*, November 1997).

Q: Now could you review some of the findings for carotenoids?

A: Much of the evidence about carotenoids' preventive effects comes from studies linking high intake and blood levels of beta carotene (and, increasingly, those of other carotenoids) to lower rates of cancer. But since other protective nutrients—including fiber and vitamin C—are present in foods rich in beta carotene, this kind of evidence doesn't necessarily mean that carotenoids protect against cancer.

In more focused studies, some carotenoids have proven effective at protecting laboratory animals against carcinogens, including chemicals, ultraviolet light and cancer cell implantation (*Lancet,* January 7, 1995). Beta carotene supplements have been shown to reduce oral leukoplakia and oral tumors in people at high risk of developing oral cancer. And since lycopene has recently been linked to lower rates of prostate and other cancers, investigators are exploring its capacities further.

VITAMIN A AND CAROTENOIDS AND THE CARDIOVASCULAR SYSTEM

Q: What effects do carotenoids and vitamin A have on the cardiovascular system?

A: Unlike the immune system, in which vitamin A and carotenoids clearly play important roles, the impact of these nutrients on the cardiovascular system is less clear. Dietary studies do suggest that foods rich in carotenoids protect the heart. But it is not yet known whether this benefit results from the antioxidant activities of carotenoids, the actions of other components of fruits and vegetables, or both.

Vitamin A and Carotenoids and Heart Disease

Q: I've heard that line before. Still, I'd like to know more about those dietary studies. What exactly did they find?

A: Primarily that people who eat the most fruits and vegetables—and, consequently, the most beta carotene and other carotenoids—are at lower risk of developing heart disease, having a heart attack or dying from heart disease, as the following studies show:

- The Nurses' Health Study and the Health Professionals Follow-up Study, widely publicized large studies that pushed vitamin E's heart-protective effects into the spotlight, also found modest heart benefits for beta carotene. The nurses' study, which followed the dietary habits and health of 87,245 women for eight years, found that women with the highest intake of beta carotene had a 22 percent lower risk of heart disease than those with the lowest intake. The health professionals' study, which followed 39,910 men for four years, found that those with the highest beta carotene intake were 25 percent less likely to suffer heart attack, stroke and other cardiovascular problems (*Contemporary Internal Medicine*, 1995).

- Italian researchers who measured the intake of foods containing beta carotene and the risk of nonfatal heart attack in women who had survived heart attacks and women without heart disease found that those who ate the fewest foods containing beta carotene had the highest risk of nonfatal heart attack (*European Journal of Epidemiology*, September 1997).

- A study analyzing data from the Iowa Women's Health Study, which followed 34,000 postmenopausal women, linked a high intake of foods rich in carotenoids, as well as those rich in vitamin A, to a slightly lower risk of death from cardiovascular disease (*New England Journal of Medicine*, May 2, 1996).

Q: Are researchers really unsure that carotenoids are the reason fruits and vegetables are so beneficial for the heart?

A: Yes. Some carotenoids are very likely to be major players in reducing risk factors such as atherosclerosis—but not necessarily when isolated from one another in supplements, or even when isolated from the other components of food that also promote cardiovascular health.

Q: I guess that makes sense, but taking supplements would be a lot easier than remembering to eat all that produce. Has anyone looked at whether beta carotene supplements benefit the heart?

A: Yes. In fact, those three long-term studies that examined the effects of beta carotene supplements on lung cancer also explored the supplements' effects on heart disease. The studies have not found that beta carotene supplements significantly lower heart disease rates. They have shown a slight or no reduction in cardiovascular disease, or even an increase in disease among men at high risk.

Q: Great—more conflicting results! Still, I guess we ought to take another look at those studies. What did they find about heart disease?

A: Let's start with the CARET trial, which, you may recall, involved more than 18,000 smokers, former smokers and workers exposed to asbestos. The study was stopped early because the group taking the active supplements was showing higher rates of some conditions than the placebo group, including 26 percent more deaths from cardiovascular disease and 17 percent more deaths overall. The researchers concluded that the combination of 25,000 I.U. of vitamin A and 30 milligrams of beta carotene had no benefit and may have had an adverse effect on cardiovascular health (*New England Journal of Medicine,* May 2, 1996).

Q: Do the researchers have any idea why the supplemented group was worse off?

A: Not yet. Because the high-risk study participants took the nutrients together, it remains unclear whether beta carotene, vitamin A or the combination was harmful to them. There was no evidence of toxicity from vitamin A, and there were no unwanted effects from beta carotene other than skin yellowing for some people, so an overdose is unlikely. The researchers note that it is possible that special conditions existed to make beta carotene act as a pro-oxidant, thus increasing LDL oxidation and promoting atherosclerosis.

Q: What about the other two studies? Did they show a connection between beta carotene supplements and heart problems?

A: For some men, yes. The initial results of the ATBC study showed that the death rates from heart disease and stroke were slightly higher among men who took beta carotene supplements than among those who did not. For the more than 27,000 (out of about 29,000) men with no history of heart attack, beta carotene supplementation (20 milligrams per day) was associated with a 6 percent increased risk of a non-fatal heart attack and a 1 percent reduced risk of fatal coronary heart disease—differences so small that the influence of chance can't be ruled out as an explanation. On the positive side, those who started the study with the highest blood levels of beta carotene had a 31 percent lower rate of nonfatal heart attack or fatal coronary heart disease than those with the lowest levels (*Archives of Internal Medicine,* March 23, 1998).

Q: What effects did beta carotene have on the men who had already had heart attacks?

A: Beta carotene had mixed effects on this group of nearly 2,000 male smokers. There were fewer nonfatal heart attacks among the men taking beta carotene than there were among those taking the placebo—33 percent fewer non-fatal heart attacks in the men taking beta carotene and 14 percent fewer in those taking beta carotene and vitamin E. But there was a 75 percent higher death rate from cardiovascular disease in the beta carotene group and a 58 percent higher death rate from cardiovascular disease in the group taking beta carotene and vitamin E compared with the placebo group. The researchers concluded that people who smoke and have had a previous heart attack should not take beta carotene or vitamin E supplements (*Lancet,* June 14, 1997).

Q: Have there been any other studies of the effects of beta carotene supplementation on people who already have cardiovascular disease?

A: Yes. In the Physicians' Health Study, the effects of beta carotene supplements (50 milligrams every other day) were examined in men with cardiovascular disease that had not yet resulted in heart attack. For the first six years of the study, the men taking beta carotene experienced 51 percent fewer major coronary events—heart attacks, strokes, sudden cardiac deaths and surgeries on clogged coronary arteries— than those taking the placebo (*Circulation,* August 1992). But the benefit all but disappeared in the next six years of the study, with a continued reduction in heart attacks in the sup- plemented men but an increase in deaths due to cardiovascular disease. The final results left researchers unsure how to inter- pret their earlier findings (*Archives of Internal Medicine,* March 23, 1998).

Q: It's interesting that those results match the ones for the smaller group in the ATBC study, with fewer nonfatal heart attacks but more deaths from cardiovascular disease. What did the Physicians' Health Study as a whole have to say about cardiovascular disease and beta carotene supplements?

A: When the results for nonsmokers, former smokers and current smokers are combined, there is virtually no difference between the rates of cardiovascular disease for men taking beta carotene and those taking a placebo. But when results are broken down according to the men's smoking status, differences emerge. Nonsmokers given beta carotene showed a combined risk of heart attack and stroke that was about 10 percent lower than the placebo group; former smokers, about 5 percent higher; and smokers, about 10 percent higher. In nonsmokers, beta carotene had no effect on the death rate from cardiovascular disease; in former and current smokers, it increased the rate by 15 percent (*New England Journal of Medicine,* May 2, 1996).

Q: Once again, smokers experience the negative effects. But what's the bottom line? What do these three studies show about cardiovascular disease and beta carotene?

A: They show that beta carotene is probably not the major player behind the heart-protective effects of fruits and vegetables.

Q: So has beta carotene been stripped of all its powers?

A: Maybe, maybe not. We did see some slight reductions in risk for nonsmokers in the Physicians' Health Study, and beta carotene has been found to have positive effects elsewhere in the body. Also, the CARET and ATBC studies did confirm that those study participants with the highest baseline blood levels of beta carotene went on to have lower rates of cancer and heart disease than those with the lowest levels, whether or not they took beta carotene supplements.

Q: What does this mean?

A: The positive association with high blood levels of beta carotene could mean, as some researchers hypothesize, that beta carotene levels are markers for the benefits of fruit and vegetable intake. It does not necessarily prove that beta carotene itself is the magic bullet. It could also mean, despite the results of studies of smokers, former smokers and asbestos workers, that beta carotene is at least slightly beneficial in those who don't smoke.

Q: Have researchers reached an overall conclusion based on all the seemingly contradictory data about beta carotene and heart disease?

A: Yes, and the conclusion is not promising. The results of large studies using beta carotene supplements show a slight reduction in risk, no reduction in risk or even a slightly increased risk of cardiovascular disease. Admittedly, the study volunteers were primarily male smokers or workers exposed to asbestos—a somewhat limited sample. Still, a review of 45 studies concludes that beta carotene has repeatedly been shown to be ineffective against cardiovascular disease (*Current Opinion in Lipidology,* December 1996). And a review of 88 research articles determined not only that beta carotene supplementation fails to decrease cardiovascular disease but also that a general recommendation for taking any antioxidant supplement as a preventive measure can't yet be made (*Prostaglandins, Leukotrienes and Essential Fatty Acids,* October 1997). Another review, this one of 37 studies of antioxidants, agrees that it would be premature to recommend widespread use of antioxidant vitamins, including beta carotene, for cardiovascular protection (*Canadian Journal of Cardiology,* October 1997).

Q: What does research into other carotenoids show? Do they play roles in cardiovascular health?

A: Some recent studies suggest that lycopene, lutein and zeaxanthin and other carotenoids may prove to be more effective than beta carotene. And we shouldn't forget that evaluations of dietary intake in large groups continue to find that foods rich in carotenoids—and high blood carotenoid levels—are linked to a lower risk of heart attack, which could support the idea of a protective effect for other carotenoids.

Heart-Protective Mechanisms of Carotenoids

Q: Do experts have any idea how carotenoids might protect the heart?

A: They have one fairly strong theory—that antioxidant carotenoids prevent the oxidation of LDL, the so-called bad cholesterol. Oxidized LDL, you may recall, is believed to lead to the development of atherosclerosis, which contributes to **coronary-artery disease** and stroke. Antioxidant carotenoids are believed to reduce the risk of atherosclerosis or lessen its severity by slowing or preventing the oxidation of LDL cholesterol.

Q: Is there any evidence that carotenoids actually do this?

A: Yes. Some studies of fruit and vegetable consumption associate higher intake with lower LDL cholesterol levels, and as we've seen, a high LDL cholesterol level can contribute to atherosclerosis.

Studies examining beta carotene's role in reducing LDL cholesterol have produced mixed results, so researchers are investigating other carotenoids. In a small Israeli study, researchers found that 60 milligrams of lycopene daily for three months resulted in a 14 percent reduction in LDL cholesterol levels in men (*Biochemical and Biophysical Research Communications,* April 28, 1997).

Q: Again, lycopene sounds promising. What about the prevention of oxidation you mentioned?

A: Some studies have found that certain carotenoids make LDL less susceptible to oxidation, preventing at least some of the first steps toward atherosclerosis. These results are not conclusive, however, because most of this research takes place in test tubes, not humans. Besides, not even all test-tube studies have found this positive effect. Some have found that under particular circumstances, some carotenoids can act as pro-oxidants, which can increase oxidative damage.

Q: **I'd still like to know more about how carotenoids may affect LDL oxidation. Could we take a look at some of the studies?**

A: Sure. Let's start with some test-tube studies. Two of these studies found protective effects for beta carotene and other carotenoids, but the third study, a two-part study that tested beta carotene in the lab and in humans, did not.

- The most recent of these studies found that the carotenoids beta carotene, canthaxanthin and zeaxanthin slowed LDL oxidation, suggesting that dietary carotenoids might help slow the progression of atherosclerosis (*FEBS Letters,* January 20, 1997).

- An earlier study of beta carotene alone also found that beta carotene interfered with LDL oxidation. The researchers suggest that previous studies finding that beta carotene did not have this effect may not have correctly prepared the beta carotene (*Acta Biochimica et Biophysica,* October 15, 1991).

- The third study had two parts, one exploring the effects of beta carotene on LDL oxidation in test tubes and another investigating its effects in people. Both parts of the study found that supplementation with beta carotene did not reduce LDL oxidation and, thus, would not help prevent atherosclerosis (*Atherosclerosis,* January 20, 1995).

Q: **That's perplexing. Have any other human studies been conducted?**

A: Yes. Let's look first at two 1997 studies. In a study published in the September 1997 *European Journal of Clinical Nutrition,* researchers gave smokers and nonsmokers a diet high in carotenoids and found that the increased carotenoid intake made LDL more resistant to oxidation for both groups, meaning that the LDL in their blood took longer to produce free radicals. These results suggest that eating more carotenoid-rich foods may reduce the risk of atherosclerosis in both smokers and nonsmokers.

In the other study, researchers at the University of Minnesota at Minneapolis analyzed blood samples and examined the arteries of people with no diagnosed cardiovascular problems to determine how blood levels of carotenoids and vitamin A affect the development of atherosclerosis. The researchers discovered that blood levels of lutein and zeaxanthin offered the strongest protection against the beginnings of atherosclerosis. Neither beta carotene nor vitamin A had significant protective effects (*Arteriosclerosis, Thrombosis and Vascular Biology*, June 1997).

Q: Why do researchers do so many studies of beta carotene if it doesn't necessarily protect against atherosclerosis?

A: The process of trial and error takes time, and some studies have found beta carotene to have a beneficial effect on LDL oxidation. But as you can see, other carotenoids may turn out to be more important in this area of cardiovascular health.

VITAMIN A AND CAROTENOIDS AND THE RESPIRATORY SYSTEM

Q: Didn't you mention that vitamin A and carotenoids have some beneficial effects on the respiratory system?

A: Yes. Beta carotene seems to protect against the lung damage caused by smoking and cystic fibrosis. And one particular retinoid reversed **emphysema** in a recent animal study. Let's look at each of these separately, starting with smoking.

Vitamin A and Carotenoids and Smoking

Q: What does smoking have to do with vitamin A and carotenoids?

A: Studies have found that smokers have lower blood levels of vitamin A and carotenoids than nonsmokers who take in the same amounts of these nutrients. These findings suggest that smoking depletes the body of these nutrients.

Q: How?

A: In part by releasing harmful free radicals into the lungs and blood. Carotenoids and other antioxidants are used up neutralizing these free radicals.

Q: So is that how beta carotene protects against lung damage, by fighting free radicals?

A: Yes. A study reported in a 1995 issue of *International Journal for Vitamin and Nutrition Research* found that low blood levels of beta carotene in smokers were associated with lower lung function. The researchers concluded that the beta carotene levels of smokers may determine how vulnerable they are to lung damage caused by oxidation. Smokers with relatively high dietary and blood levels of antioxidants have been found less likely than those with low levels to develop two diseases that oxidative damage can help cause—lung cancer and atherosclerosis.

Q: But haven't you said that higher blood levels of beta carotene aren't necessarily responsible for a lower incidence of disease?

A: We have. But studies do suggest that antioxidants, including beta carotene, benefit the lungs. In one such study, a group of researchers evaluated whether a small group of smokers and nonsmokers taking 24 milligrams of beta carotene, 800 I.U. of vitamin E and 1,000 milligrams of vitamin C daily had a lower exhaled ethane output. The level of exhaled ethane output indicates how much lipid peroxidation is occurring in the body. (Lipid peroxidation, as you may recall, is the process of fats interacting with oxygen to create potentially harmful free radicals. Not only can this process start the chain reaction that can lead to clogged arteries, but it can also contribute to lung damage and reduced lung function.) The researchers found that exhaled ethane output decreased by an average of 29 percent in smokers taking the supplements. This decrease translated into improvements in lung function, leading the researchers to conclude that antioxidants may lessen smoking-related lung injuries (*Chest,* July 1996).

Vitamin A and Carotenoids and Lung Disease

Q: You said earlier that beta carotene also seems to protect the lungs from damage caused by cystic fibrosis. What is cystic fibrosis, and what does it have to do with the lungs?

A: Cystic fibrosis is a hereditary disease that affects the secretion of fluids from many glands, making these fluids abnormally thick. In the lungs, this thick mucus clogs the airways and allows bacteria to multiply. This situation causes severe lung inflammation and lung injury. The amount of lipid peroxidation increases, worsening these lung problems.

Q: How does beta carotene fit into this equation?

A: Beta carotene is an antioxidant and, as such, may help reduce lipid peroxidation in the lungs, thus reducing lung damage in people with cystic fibrosis.

Q: Does beta carotene reduce lipid peroxidation in people with cystic fibrosis?

A: It appears to. One small study of children with and without cystic fibrosis found very low blood levels of beta carotene in those with the illness. When these children took about 4 milligrams of beta carotene three times a day, their blood levels of beta carotene rose, and their levels of malondialdehyde, a marker of lipid peroxidation, dropped. The researchers determined that beta carotene deficiency contributes to lipid peroxidation in children with cystic fibrosis and that beta carotene supplementation reduces lipid peroxidation (*American Journal of Clinical Nutrition,* July 1996).

Swiss researchers also found low blood levels of beta carotene in people with cystic fibrosis. They gave beta carotene supplements to people with and without the disease. Not only did blood levels of beta carotene increase in all participants, but after three months, differences in the amount and rate of lipid peroxidation had disappeared between the people with the disease and those with healthy lungs (*Free Radical Biology and Medicine,* May 1995).

Q: Would beta carotene help with just about any lung disease, then?

A: It's tempting to say yes, this reduction in oxidative reactions would probably benefit just about anyone with a respiratory illness. But then again, the results from the CARET and ATBC studies regarding people with lung damage from smoking and asbestos exposure suggest that beta carotene can't always be assumed to act as an antioxidant. We shouldn't forget its pro-oxidant potential.

Q: You mentioned earlier that a retinoid can help with emphysema. What is emphysema, and how does that retinoid help?

A: Emphysema is a disease that damages the **alveoli**, tiny air sacs in the lungs, causing narrowed airways and restricting breathing. Until recently, its damage was believed to be irreversible. But in a groundbreaking study by researchers at Georgetown University, a retinoid succeeded in reversing emphysema in rats. In an earlier study, these researchers had found that all-trans-retinoic acid stimulated alveoli growth in the lungs of healthy rats by 50 percent. When they gave all-trans-retinoic acid to rats with emphysema, the number and size of alveoli, along with the volume of the lungs, returned to normal (*Lancet,* June 7, 1997). Further testing is needed to determine if the retinoid will help people with emphysema.

VITAMIN A AND CAROTENOIDS AND THE EYES

Q: What can vitamin A and the carotenoids do for the eyes?

A: Vitamin A helps maintain the epithelial tissue that lines the eye and is used by the eye in its functions, including those that enable us to see in darkness. Night blindness is an early sign of a vitamin A deficiency.

Further, the carotenoids lutein and zeaxanthin are present in the macula, a tiny area at the center of the retina. Studies suggest that these antioxidants may help prevent **cataracts**, which result from the clouding of the eye's transparent lens. Cataracts block light from reaching the retina, leading to blindness. This clouding is thought to result from oxidation in the eye, often caused by sunlight.

Q: What evidence is there that lutein and zeaxanthin may help prevent cataracts?

A: In a 1997 study at Arizona State University, researchers measured levels of lutein and zeaxanthin in the retinas and the amount of lens clouding in men and women ages 24 to 82. As expected, they found that the amount of lens clouding increased with age. But they also found that older study participants with low levels of lutein and zeaxanthin had more lens clouding than older participants with high levels, indicating that intake of these nutrients may help slow age-related increases in lens clouding, which can lead to cataracts (*Optometry and Vision Science*, July 1997).

Q: I know that lutein and zeaxanthin are antioxidants, but do they function as antioxidants in the eye?

A: Yes. A study by the U.S. Department of Agriculture found by-products of lutein and zeaxanthin's antioxidant function in the human retina, showing that these carotenoids probably help to protect the macula against light damage. This protection may play a vital role in preventing both cataracts and age-related macular degeneration, the breakdown of the macula that causes a gradual loss of vision (*Investigative Ophthalmology and Visual Science*, August 1997).

Q: Do lutein and zeaxanthin help protect against macular degeneration?

A: They appear to. Several studies in the mid-1980s found that people eating the fewest fruits and vegetables had the highest incidence of macular degeneration. Researchers initially attributed this benefit to beta carotene, but a 1994 study conducted by Harvard Medical School and several leading eye institutions reexamined food intake data from those earlier studies and found that a high intake of leafy green vegetables— not the orange and yellow ones that are highest in beta carotene—had led to the lower rate of macular degeneration.

The researchers reported that people eating greens two to four times a week had 50 percent less chance of macular degeneration than those eating greens less than once a month. People eating greens five or more times a week had an even lower risk. The researchers reasoned that a protective effect for lutein and zeaxanthin seems very likely since they are the dominant carotenoids in leafy greens, form the yellow pigment in the macula and filter out the visible blue light that can cause oxidation (*Journal of the American Medical Association*, November 9, 1994).

Q: Does that mean beta carotene doesn't help?

A: Maybe. One study of people with and without macular degeneration found no evidence of a protective effect from beta carotene (*American Journal of Ophthalmology*, December 1997). But a study focusing only on people with macular degeneration found that supplementation with a multivitamin and mineral supplement that included 20,000 I.U. of beta carotene significantly slowed the progression of the disease (*Journal of the American Optometric Association*, January 1996).

VITAMIN A AND CAROTENOIDS AND THE SKIN

Q: Isn't vitamin A used to treat skin conditions other than cancer?

A: Yes. Vitamin A has been used since the early 1940s to treat acne. The vitamin promotes healthy skin growth and reduces inflammation, which both results from and can worsen acne. Two drugs made from vitamin A are tretinoin, which comes in creams such as Retin-A and Renova and has been used for a long time to treat acne, and isotretinoin (Accutane), which is taken orally to treat severe acne.

Q: Doesn't Retin-A help get rid of wrinkles?

A: Somewhat. News that Retin-A could reduce wrinkles was released in 1988, generating much excitement. But according to the newsletter *Consumer Reports on Health* (February 1998), a review of the research on antiaging creams published in the *Medical Letter on Drugs and Therapeutics* found that skin creams containing tretinoin, such as Retin-A and Renova, have only a modest effect on fine wrinkles and age spots and can cause stinging, burning and redness.

Q: Can vitamin A help with any skin problems besides wrinkles, acne and the precancerous and cancerous conditions we looked at earlier?

A: Yes. The medical world has long known that vitamin A is beneficial to the skin, and it is far beyond the initial phases of research into using forms of vitamin A for skin problems. Retinoids called etretrinate (Tegison) and acitretin (Soriatane) are used regularly and successfully by doctors to treat many skin diseases, including psoriasis (a chronic, recurring disease causing bumps and raised, flaky patches of skin) and related problems. Isotretinoin (Accutane) is used successfully for seborrheic dermatitis (an inflammation that causes scales on the skin, usually on the scalp and face), rosacea (a persistent skin disorder that produces redness, tiny pimples and broken blood vessels, usually in the central part of the face) and acneiform dermatosis, as well as severe acne. And the retinoid creams we mentioned, in addition to offering relief from acne and some signs of aging, are used to treat disorders of skin pigmentation (*Drugs,* March 1997).

Q: Do carotenoids have any known benefits for the skin?

A: Skin applications and oral doses of beta carotene have been shown to lessen skin damage caused by ultraviolet light, which causes tissue damage from free radicals and is a major cause of the signs of aging. Exposure to ultraviolet light can also suppress the immune system. Several studies suggest that beta carotene may help protect against these immune-suppressing effects, which may be factors in skin cancer. A recent German study showed that beta carotene protects against damage caused by ultraviolet-A (but not ultraviolet-B) rays and also showed that one form of beta carotene (13-cis-beta carotene) inhibits the oxidative damage that leads to inflammation in skin cells. The researchers found these effects in test tubes and in people (*Inflammation Research,* October 1997). And in a small study, healthy women who took 30 milligrams of beta carotene per day and used sunscreen experienced less redness when their skin was exposed to sunlight than women who took a placebo and used sunscreen (*European Journal of Dermatology*, 1996).

OTHER VITAMIN A AND CAROTENOID USES

Q: Are there any other health problems that vitamin A and the carotenoids might help prevent or fight?

A: Yes. A vitamin A deficiency may lead to a higher rate of mother-to-child transmission of human immunodeficiency virus (HIV), the virus that causes AIDS, and beta carotene may help boost immunity in people with HIV. Carotenoids in the diet may help prevent **rheumatoid arthritis**. And vitamin A is often given to premature infants to prevent lung problems, although its effectiveness is unproven. Let's look first at possible benefits for those infected with HIV.

Vitamin A and Carotenoids and Human Immunodeficiency Virus

Q: What does vitamin A have to do with HIV?

A: A vitamin A deficiency damages immunity, so the body can't fight the virus as well. A review of the current research by investigators at Johns Hopkins University has special significance for pregnant women with HIV: Those who are deficient in vitamin A have higher levels of the virus in their blood and in their breast milk than those with adequate levels of vitamin A, reflecting immune system damage (*Acta Paediatrica, Supplement*, June 1997). These women may be more likely to transmit the virus to their infants. Studies are under way to see whether giving daily nutrient supplements that include vitamin A to pregnant women with HIV who are deficient in vitamin A will reduce mother-to-infant transmission of the virus.

Q: **Didn't you say that vitamin A deficiencies are seen mostly in developing countries?**

A: Yes, and some of the research on this topic has been done in Africa, possibly including women with inadequate intake of many nutrients. But results of two studies of urban American women were released in 1997. One found no relationship between blood vitamin A levels and maternal HIV transmission and no level of vitamin A low enough to qualify as a deficiency (*Journal of Acquired Immune Deficiency Syndrome,* April 1, 1997). The other study found that some women with HIV had severe vitamin A deficiencies and that these deficiencies were in fact associated with mother-to-infant transmission of HIV (*AIDS,* March 1997).

Q: **What about women transmitting HIV to sexual partners—has any research been done on that?**

A: Yes. One of the recent studies, conducted by the University of Washington, looked at whether women deficient in vitamin A shed more HIV-infected cells from the cervix and vagina than those with adequate vitamin A levels. The researchers found that women with low-normal, moderately deficient and severely deficient vitamin A status shed five to 13 times more HIV-infected cells than women with normal vitamin A status. This means they would be more likely to pass the disease to sexual partners (*Lancet,* September 27, 1997).

Q: **Have vitamin A or carotenoids been found to have any positive effects on other aspects of the health of people with HIV?**

A: Yes and no. One recent study at Johns Hopkins University sought to discover whether vitamin A could affect HIV replication (the reproduction of the virus). HIV-infected users of injection drugs were given either a single dose of 200,000 I.U. of vitamin A or a placebo. The supplementation had no significant effect on the amount of the virus in their blood or on certain immune system fighters (*Journal of Infectious Diseases,* March 1998).

Yet two earlier short-term studies in which people with HIV were given either beta carotene or a placebo found that those who took a very high dose of beta carotene—180 milligrams per day—had a significant rise in their levels of certain immune system cells, including the ones measured in the Johns Hopkins study. These studies suggest that high-dose supplementation with beta carotene may improve immunity in HIV-infected people, possibly leading to less vulnerability to other infections and to a delay of the progression to AIDS (*Medical Tribune,* February 25, 1993, and *Journal of Acquired Immune Deficiency Syndrome,* December 1993).

Q: Have more recent studies confirmed those results?

A: A 1997 study at the Oregon Health Sciences University did not. Researchers found no significant differences in several immune system measures between the supplemented and placebo groups in a long-term test of beta carotene supplements. Participants with HIV took either 60 milligrams of beta carotene or a placebo three times daily for three months. In addition, all participants were given a multivitamin supplement, which the researchers admit may have masked any difference between the two groups by boosting immunity in both. However, taking into account the smaller size and shorter terms of the earlier studies showing a benefit along with the results of their study, the researchers do not recommend high doses of beta carotene for people infected with HIV (*AIDS,* August 1996).

Carotenoids and
Rheumatoid Arthritis

Q: Do carotenoids benefit people with rheumatoid arthritis?

A: Possibly. A study found a promising connection between high blood levels of beta carotene and a lower risk of rheumatoid arthritis, a disease in which the immune system fights against its own tissue, causing inflammation and joint damage that can make it difficult to move areas such as the knuckles and ankles. But we know by now that this result could mean that some factor *associated* with beta carotene, and not beta carotene itself, is the helpful substance. Still, the study does suggest a link and does open paths for further research.

Q: How could beta carotene help prevent rheumatoid arthritis?

A: The fluid in the lining of inflamed joints contains the products of considerable oxidative damage, and an antioxidant could prevent some of those oxidative reactions from occurring. People with rheumatoid arthritis have lower than normal blood levels of beta carotene, which might indicate that their stores are being used up in fighting those oxidative reactions.

Q: So this study looked at blood levels of beta carotene?

A: That's right. Researchers at Johns Hopkins University looked at blood samples taken from more than 20,000 people in 1974, then determined who had developed rheumatoid arthritis in the next 15 years. The 1974 blood levels of beta carotene among people who had developed the condition were 29 percent lower than levels among those who hadn't. The lead researcher, George Comstock, M.D., was quoted as saying, "People should interpret the results to mean that they should eat more fruits and vegetables" (*Tufts University Health and Nutrition Letter,* September 1997).

Q: We've heard that recommendation a few times, haven't we?

A: We certainly have. And research does back it up!

Vitamin A and Premature Infants

Q: Does vitamin A help premature infants avoid lung problems?

A: Possibly. Many intensive care units do give vitamin A supplements to premature infants to prevent lung damage and boost immunity because enough research suggests it could benefit these infants. But one research review could report only that the rise in blood vitamin A levels from supplementation may help lower death rates in these infants and that the supplementation is safe (*European Journal of Clinical Nutrition,* July 1996). And a small Italian study that gave premature babies 1,000 I.U. of vitamin A intravenously for their first 28 days of life found no association between blood concentrations of the vitamin and health. While the researchers wrote that the supplementation caused no detectable negative effects, they also noted that the effectiveness of this treatment hasn't yet been adequately proven (*International Journal of Clinical Pharmacology Therapy,* August 1996).

PUTTING IT ALL TOGETHER

Q: We've looked at lots of results, but I'm still not sure what to think. Some of the research shows important benefits, and other research doesn't. How can I figure out which results to believe and whether to take supplements when there may not yet be enough evidence?

A: Keep up with the research in areas that concern you. Remember, too, that some studies are more reliable than others. The most reliable studies are those that seek to determine the effects of vitamin A or carotenoid supplements in a group of people and compare these results with those found in a group taking a placebo. While animal studies and studies of dietary intake provide interesting findings, they can't provide specific recommendations for the intake of a single nutrient for people. Then again, you might not want to think in terms of single nutrients. As we've seen, eating lots of fruits and vegetables is an excellent way to gain protection from many diseases.

Q: But what if I'm at risk for a particular condition that some research indicates might be helped by a beta carotene supplement? Should I take the supplement even if all the research doesn't show the benefit?

A: Because research doesn't provide all the answers, you will have to make your own choices about supplementation. But keeping track of research findings as they are released can help you make informed choices. In the next chapter, we look at some practical aspects of vitamin A and the carotenoids, and this information might help make your choices a little easier.

3 WHAT ELSE DO I NEED TO KNOW?

Q: I'm impressed with all of the ways carotenoids and vitamin A might help prevent and treat illness. Even if they are proven effective in just a few of those cases, these nutrients are still vital to our general health, right?

A: Definitely. As we said in chapter 1, vitamin A helps maintain crucial bodily functions such as the immune system, and it helps keep epithelial tissue healthy throughout the body. Children's survival and growth depends on their getting enough vitamin A, among other nutrients. And carotenoids also play vital roles throughout our bodies, whether as antioxidants or through other functions. Eating fruits and vegetables, which abound in carotenoids, is clearly an effective way to help prevent heart disease and cancer, along with other conditions such as cataracts, macular degeneration and perhaps even rheumatoid arthritis.

Carotenoid precursors of vitamin A are present in the following herbs: alfalfa, borage leaves, burdock root, cayenne (capsicum), chickweed, eyebright, fennel seed, hops, horsetail, kelp, lemongrass, mullein, nettle, oat straw, paprika, parsley, peppermint, plantain, raspberry leaf, red clover, rose hips, sage, uva ursi, violet leaves, watercress and yellow dock.

DOSAGE

Q: How much vitamin A and carotenoids do we need to stay healthy and prevent disease?

A: Actually, you're asking two questions. To give our bodies the amount of vitamin A they need to keep us healthy, we need to get the Recommended Dietary Allowance (RDA) for our gender and age-group. These amounts prevent deficiency symptoms in most healthy people. But to prevent disease, we may need to get more than what it takes to prevent deficiency. As for carotenoids, no RDAs have been set, although they are clearly beneficial nutrients.

Q: Do the RDAs tell us the minimum amounts that most healthy people need to get every day?

A: Yes and no. The RDAs are levels of nutrient intake— whether gotten from foods, supplements or a combination—that the National Academy of Sciences' Food and Nutrition Board believes to be adequate to meet the known nutrient needs of most healthy people. But since fat-soluble vitamins such as vitamin A are stored in the liver and fatty tissues, you can take in more on one day and less on the next and not suffer a shortage.

Q: What are the RDAs of vitamin A?

A: Our need depends in part on body weight, so the recommended amounts for men and women reflect the weight difference that usually exists between them, with the women's RDA set at 80 percent of the men's. The RDA of vitamin A is 800 RE for women and 1,000 RE for men. The chart that follows gives the daily RDAs for both genders and all age-groups.

Recommended Dietary Allowances of Vitamin A

Category	Age	Amount (RE)
Infants	0-6 months	375
	6-12 months	375
Children	1-3 years	400
	4-6 years	500
	7-10 years	700
Men	11+ years	1,000
Women	11+ years	800
	Pregnant	800
	Lactating (1st 6 months)	1,300
	Lactating (2nd 6 months)	1,200

Q: **Can you refresh my memory about what RE stands for?**

A: Of course. RE stands for retinol equivalent, and retinol is a common form of vitamin A found in many foods. As you may remember, some carotenoids can be converted to vitamin A. The retinol equivalent was created so that we can talk about the amount of retinol provided, whether by retinol itself or by a carotenoid that can be converted to retinol in the body.

Q: **A lot of the studies we looked at listed vitamin A in I.U. Can you remind me what an I.U. is?**

A: Sure. I.U. stands for international unit, a unit of measurement that researchers use to quantify both vitamin A and vitamin E.

Q: What's the equivalent in I.U. of the RDA of vitamin A?

A: The vitamin A requirement of 800 RE for women translates to 4,000 I.U., and the requirement of 1,000 RE for men translates to 5,000 I.U., as we noted in chapter 1.

Q: And how about for beta carotene—didn't you give those values earlier?

A: Yes. Although there is no RDA for beta carotene, scientists have figured out the amount of beta carotene needed for the body to create the equivalent of both an RE and an I.U. of retinol. To get the equivalent of the women's RDA of retinol, you'd need to take in 800 RE, or 8,000 I.U., of beta carotene. To get the equivalent of the men's RDA of retinol, you'd need to take in 1,000 RE, or 10,000 I.U., of beta carotene.

> **Women's RDA of retinol:**
> *800 RE or 4,000 I.U.*
>
> **Women's beta carotene equivalent:**
> *800 RE, 8,000 I.U. or 5 milligrams*
>
> **Men's RDA of retinol:**
> *1,000 RE or 5,000 I.U.*
>
> **Men's beta carotene equivalent:**
> *1,000 RE, 10,000 I.U. or 6 milligrams*

Q: Didn't the studies we looked at refer to beta carotene in milligrams?

A: Yes, they did. Here are the equivalents of the RDA figures for beta carotene in milligrams. One milligram of beta carotene equals about 1,700 I.U. So 8,000 and 10,000 I.U. of beta carotene equal about 5 milligrams and 6 milligrams, respectively.

Q: That doesn't sound like much. What dosages of beta carotene supplements did the studies use?

A: Many of the studies of beta carotene we looked at used supplements of about 20 to 30 milligrams daily—amounts that someone eating the recommended five to nine servings of fruits and vegetables per day would be likely to get.

Q: What are the equivalents of the vitamin A RDA for other carotenoids that can be converted to retinol?

A: Equivalents of retinol for other carotenoid precursors are not widely known, if they are known at all.

Q: Did you say that the RDAs are being revised?

A: Yes. The Food and Nutrition Board is in the process of reviewing the latest research on each nutrient for which it issues requirements. It is taking into consideration not just the amount of each nutrient needed to avoid deficiency but also the amount needed to decrease the risk of chronic diseases such as heart disease and cancer. These revised RDAs will become part of a new set of recommendations known as Dietary Reference Intakes (DRIs).

Q: When will the DRIs for vitamin A be released?

A: The board hopes to arrive at DRIs for all essential nutrients by the year 2000, but it hasn't yet given interim dates for the release of information on each nutrient.

Q: In the meantime, how can I know how much vitamin A to get to reduce my risk of chronic diseases and reap the vitamin's full benefits?

A: Until the new recommendations are released, you might want to follow the existing RDAs. Don't forget that vitamin A does get stored in the body and can cause toxicity. Since some people react negatively to a single dose of vitamin A as low as 20,000 I.U., and since a regular dose of 50,000 I.U. may cause toxicity after a few months, few people recommend regularly taking much more than the RDA. The exception is if a doctor prescribes it because you have difficulty absorbing the vitamin or you are being treated for a serious illness and a form of vitamin A is being used as a medication.

You may have noticed that few studies use vitamin A itself as a supplement; instead, they use beta carotene. Even for people with cystic fibrosis, who generally have chronic vitamin A deficiencies, recent studies have tested the effectiveness of beta carotene, not vitamin A, at reversing those deficiencies. As noted earlier, beta carotene supplementation has no known chance of causing toxicity, and the body converts it to vitamin A as needed.

Q: Is there an optimal amount of beta carotene I should try to get every day?

A: Not exactly. Eating at least five servings of fruits and vegetables per day will give you plenty of beta carotene. As for supplementation, no recommendations have been made by major health organizations for beta carotene supplementation. While even high-dose supplements appear to be safe for many people and may help with certain medical conditions, their benefits over fruit and vegetable intake for

> *The following fruits and vegetables contain high amounts of beta carotene: dried apricots (5 milligrams per ounce), dried peaches (3 milligrams per ounce), carrots and sweet potatoes (2 milligrams per ounce).*

generally healthy people haven't been proven. And some studies have shown possible harmful effects from moderate beta carotene supplementation for people at high risk of getting certain conditions.

On the plus side, since beta carotene is converted to vitamin A only when that nutrient is needed, it won't cause an overdose of vitamin A. If you eat plenty of fruits and vegetables and have no difficulties absorbing fat-soluble vitamins, you should be in no danger of having a vitamin A deficiency.

Q: Could you list the symptoms of a vitamin A deficiency again?

A: Sure. The first symptom of a vitamin A deficiency is usually night blindness. Eye symptoms grow worse if the deficiency continues, and an extreme deficiency can lead to the permanent loss of eyesight. Other symptoms of a vitamin A deficiency include skin disorders (such as hard, pigmented goose bumps), deficient mucus secretions, dry mouth, loss of appetite and reduced resistance to infection. As we noted, children need the vitamin to help them grow, so their deficiency symptoms can also include stunted growth, crooked teeth and improper bone formation.

Q: Didn't you say in chapter 1 that certain people are at increased risk of a vitamin A deficiency?

A: Yes. People with diseases that affect the intestines' ability to absorb fat have difficulty absorbing fat-soluble vitamins such as vitamin A. These diseases include cystic fibrosis and celiac disease. Other people at increased risk include the institutionalized elderly, alcoholics and the critically ill. Also, people who follow very low fat diets may not be taking in enough fat to allow the body to absorb fat-soluble vitamins, including vitamin A.

Q: Are any people at increased risk of a carotenoid deficiency?

A: Yes. Many conditions can put people at risk of having low blood concentrations of beta carotene. These include rheumatoid arthritis and cystic fibrosis. Smoking and drinking also stress the body and can lead to lower beta carotene levels. Those with severe burns or other injuries may also become deficient since the healing of these injuries uses up lots of beta carotene and other antioxidants.

Q: Didn't you say that people's lifestyles can influence their blood levels of carotenoids and vitamin A?

A: We certainly did. Exercise, smoking, alcohol use, infections and exposure to air pollution, among other things, can increase oxidative stress. This increases the body's use of antioxidants, including carotenoids, possibly leading to lower-than-normal blood levels of some carotenoids. Smokers have been shown to have lower blood levels of beta carotene and retinol than nonsmokers, and those who drink a lot of alcohol have been shown to have lower blood levels of beta carotene but higher levels of retinol.

Q: Does smoking lower blood levels of all carotenoids?

A: No. In some studies, lycopene levels have not been lower in smokers; nor does this particular carotenoid appear to be affected by drinking. Instead, the most significant factor for lycopene levels is age, with levels usually dropping as people grow older.

However, a study in which human blood was exposed to cigarette smoke found that lycopene was the carotenoid most quickly destroyed by the smoke (*American Journal of Clinical Nutrition*, October 1997).

TOXICITY

Q: Does anyone need **megadoses** of vitamin A?

A: That depends in part on what you mean by the word megadose. Many people use the word to mean a large dose. But according to its scientific definition, a megadose is a dose of 10 times the RDA or more. For vitamin A, that would mean 8,000 RE (or 40,000 I.U.) for women and 10,000 RE (or 50,000 I.U.) for men. As we've pointed out, taking this amount would not be a good idea for most people because taking about 50,000 I.U. of vitamin A daily over time can lead to a toxic overload of vitamin A in the body. And some people react negatively to lower doses.

In addition, vitamin A can cause malformation in developing embryos. (Keep in mind, however, that adequate vitamin A is vital for the healthy development of the embryo, so pregnant women should aim to get their RDA.) Contraception is absolutely essential for women who could become pregnant during and even soon after medical treatment with a retinoid taken orally, and even prescription retinoid creams are not recommended for women who could become pregnant because their safety has not yet been proven (*Archives de Pediatrie,* September 1997). Anyone taking a retinoid drug should have frequent checkups to ensure that she hasn't built up a toxic level of vitamin A.

Q: Could you remind me again about the signs of vitamin A toxicity?

A: Early signs of toxicity include fatigue, nausea, vomiting, headache, vertigo, blurred vision, loss of muscle coordination and loss of body hair. Signs of long-term excessive intake of vitamin A can include headache, flaky skin, spleen enlargement, bone thickening and joint pain. Anyone who experiences these symptoms while taking vitamin A should consult his physician. And anyone taking a vitamin A drug as a medical treatment should be instructed as to what signs of toxicity to look for and should remain alert to their possible appearance. If you are taking the acne drug isotretinoin (Accutane), for example, you should watch for possible effects on your mental state. A recent article in the journal *Lancet* (March 7, 1998) points out that the U.S. Food and Drug Administration has just required that labeling for isotretinoin contain a warning that depression, psychosis, suicidal thoughts and suicide may be caused by the drug. Some people taking the drug have experienced an increase in these symptoms, which disappeared when they halted the treatment.

Q: Do megadoses of beta carotene cause toxicity?

A: So far, very large amounts have not been found to cause toxicity in animals or humans. They can cause carotenemia, a harmless condition characterized by a yellow tint to the skin. But on the other hand, high doses can't be assumed to have positive effects.

As you may remember from chapter 2, some studies suggest that the actions of beta carotene are not entirely predictable, especially in smokers who drink a lot of alcohol. A recent article examining the results from studies of large groups taking beta carotene supplements concludes that smokers should avoid using high-dose beta carotene supplements (*Nutrition Reviews,* October 1997).

Q: What amount qualifies as a high dose of beta carotene?

A: The studies that found negative effects for some smokers used dosages of 20 to 30 milligrams daily, much lower than a megadose. A megadose of beta carotene— 10 times the RDA—would be 8,000 RE, 80,000 I.U. or 50 milligrams for women and 10,000 RE, 100,000 I.U. or 60 milligrams for men.

Q: Are megadoses of beta carotene beneficial?

A: With a few possible exceptions, the benefits of mega-doses of beta carotene haven't been firmly established. Results have often been mixed, with some studies of people with a certain condition benefiting from a megadose and others failing to show this benefit. We saw this inconsistency when we looked at the studies using megadoses for people with HIV infection.

DRUG INTERACTIONS

Q: Do any drugs negatively interact with vitamin A?

A: Yes. Many drugs made from vitamin A should not be taken with supplemental vitamin A since the risk of toxicity increases with additional intake. These drugs include the acne medicine isotretinoin (Accutane). Other drugs can affect the absorption of fats and fat-soluble vitamins, so they can cause a deficiency of vitamin A by impeding absorption. Drugs with this effect include a class of cholesterol medications known as bile acid sequestrants (cholestyramine [Questran] and colestipol hydrochloride [Colestid], for example) and mineral oil laxatives, if they are used regularly.

Q: Do any drugs have a negative effect on carotenoids?

A: Yes. Some drugs and other substances lower blood levels and absorption of carotenoids.
A recent study found significantly below normal blood levels of beta carotene in women ages 25 to 44 who use oral contraceptives, although no such effect occurred in women ages 18 to 24 (*Veris,* March 1998). In another study, the cholesterol drugs probucol (Lorelco) and cholestyramine decreased blood

levels of beta carotene and lycopene, with reductions of 30 to 40 percent (*Arteriosclerosis, Thrombosis and Vascular Biology,* August 1995). And although it is not a drug, the fat substitute olestra (Olean) bears mentioning; a four-month study by Procter and Gamble showed that blood levels of beta carotene, alpha carotene, lycopene, lutein and zeaxanthin were all reduced by about 25 percent in people who ate 18 grams of olestra per day (*Journal of Nutrition,* August 1997).

As for absorption, the drug colchicine (ColBENEMID), which is used to treat gout, may impair the absorption of beta carotene.

NUTRIENT INTERACTIONS

Q: Do vitamin A or carotenoids interact with other vitamins and minerals in any way?

A: Possibly. Until recently, researchers believed that supplementation with beta carotene lowered blood levels of vitamin E, but current studies involving large groups of people have not found this effect. And since zinc is necessary for the transport of vitamin A from the liver to the rest of the body, a zinc deficiency has been found to impede the body's ability to make use of vitamin A.

Researchers are also examining the effects of carotenoid supplements on blood levels of other carotenoids. But they can't yet make generalizations about these influences because results have been so inconsistent and individual variations so wide in the many studies exploring this issue (*American Journal of Clinical Nutrition,* February 1998).

SUPPLEMENTS

Q: Speaking of supplements, I'm thinking of taking a supplement to make sure I'm getting enough vitamin A and carotenoids. What's available?

A: Quite a lot. You can get individual supplements of vitamin A, beta carotene, lycopene and lutein in a range of brands and dosages. They are also available in combination with other nutrients, whether as part of a multivitamin and mineral supplement, a supplement of mixed carotenoids or a formula intended to target a particular problem or maintain a specific part of the body.

Q: I'm not very familiar with multivitamin and mineral supplements. What vitamins and minerals do they contain and in what amounts?

A: These supplements vary widely. Most contain some but not all of the nutrients for which RDAs have been established. Some provide the full RDA of each nutrient listed, but many do not. Sometimes the more expensive individual nutrients in a multivitamin and mineral supplement are provided in smaller amounts. And some multivitamin and mineral supplements include minerals, herbs and other nutrients for which no RDAs have been established.

Q: What type of multivitamin and mineral supplement do nutrition experts recommend?

A: Actually, not all nutrition experts recommend taking nutritional supplements; instead, they advise that people eat a nutritious diet. But many do believe that a multivitamin and mineral supplement can help fill in occasional gaps in a good diet. These people generally suggest a supplement that provides 100 percent of the RDAs of those nutrients that have RDAs.

Q: Am I likely to get the RDA of vitamin A or beta carotene in a multivitamin and mineral supplement?

A: That depends on the supplement. For vitamin A, some supplements provide up to 25,000 I.U., which is five times the men's RDA of 1,000 RE, while others provide the RDA or slightly less. For carotenoids, no RDAs have been established, but amounts in individual and mixed supplements also range widely.

Q: You mentioned supplements that contain a mix of carotenoids or nutrients including carotenoids. Can you tell me more about them?

A: Sure. These supplements, which usually come in capsules, are a recent addition to the nutrient market. Some provide a mix of carotenoids, such as lutein and zeaxanthin, lycopene, beta carotene, alpha carotene and cryptoxanthin. Others contain nutrients intended to help a certain part of the body, such as the eyes; thus far, products for the eyes include lutein but not its partner, zeaxanthin. While these supplements rarely list sources for each carotenoid, they do list the ingredients forming the base of their formulas, such as pumpkin, tomato, spinach, carrot and/or broccoli concentrates. Beta carotene is also included in some supplements containing a mix of antioxidants, such as beta carotene along with vitamins C and E.

Q: I'd like to know more about individual supplements of vitamin A and carotenoids. In what forms are they available, and what sources do they use?

A: Vitamin A comes in capsules and pills. The vitamin A in capsules is usually the fat-soluble form derived from fish liver oil. The pills usually contain a water-soluble form of vitamin A called **retinyl palmitate**, which is created both naturally and synthetically and is considered preferable for people who have difficulty absorbing fats. You can also get vitamin A from cod-liver oil, which contains 4,600 I.U. of vitamin A per teaspoon. Cod-liver oil comes in a liquid form (as an oil) or in capsules.

As for individual carotenoids, they come mostly in capsules, and their sources are not always listed. If no other source is listed, the vegetable listed as the base may be the carotenoid source. Lutein, lycopene and beta carotene are available individually. Lutein may be derived from marigolds and lycopene from tomatoes. Beta carotene is usually derived from either a marine algae called dunialiella salina or carrot oil.

Q: Is there any difference between natural and synthetic vitamin A?

A: Yes. Natural vitamin A is derived from natural sources, often from fish liver oil, while synthetic vitamin A, like other synthetic vitamins, is made by combining organic molecules from an array of substances. But just because it's not called natural, synthetic vitamin A is not necessarily inferior to the natural form. If a vitamin bottle says the supplement contains 400 RE of retinol, this means that the activity of the retinol it contains is 400 RE, whether its source is synthetic or natural. Still, fish liver oil may contain other nutrients besides vitamin A, potentially offering benefits beyond those provided by a synthetic supplement.

Q: How can I tell if the supplement I'm buying is natural or synthetic?

A: A source may be listed on the label. If no source is listed, you could write to the manufacturer or choose a brand that lists the source.

Q: Is it best to get my vitamin A from capsules, from pills or as liquid from cod-liver oil?

A: This is mostly a matter of preference, though as we said, you may get additional nutrients from fish oil, whether you take it as a capsule or a liquid. If you have a hard time swallowing pills, you may prefer to take the liquid oil, which comes in several flavors. But if you find the oil hard to swallow, you may prefer capsules. And as we indicated, if you have difficulty absorbing fats, you'd probably be better off with pills of retinyl palmitate, a water-soluble form of vitamin A.

Q: We've looked at several ways of measuring vitamin A and beta carotene—I.U., RE, milligrams. How do I interpret these different measurements on vitamin bottles?

A: If your bottle lists beta carotene in I.U., RE or milligrams, compare the amount with the RDA equivalents of beta carotene, which we've listed on page 94. If the bottle lists retinol in I.U. or RE, use the retinol RDA figures provided. If it lists a combined vitamin A content from retinol and beta carotene, you won't be able to tell how much you're getting in each form unless it also lists the percentage coming from each.

Q: Is a store brand as good as other brands?

A: It may be. Many store brands are similar in formulation to brand-name vitamins, but they usually cost less. Compare labels to see if the products are comparable. And if a manufacturer claims its product is more readily absorbed or better balanced but the label doesn't explain why and you would like to know, ask the company to send you information on the research that backs up its claims.

Q: Speaking of absorption, how can I tell if I'm buying good-quality supplements and whether the supplements will dissolve properly and be absorbed?

A: Look for the letters U.S.P. on the label. This means the supplement meets manufacturing standards set by the U.S. Pharmacopoeia, an independent, nonprofit organization that evaluates nutritional supplements (along with other products) in the United States. For supplements, the U.S. Pharmacopoeia tests how well the supplement dissolves, among other measures of quality.

You can help your body absorb many of the nutrients in a supplement by taking it at the end of a meal. The digestive juices stimulated by the food will help your body break down and absorb the supplement. And when taking a fat-soluble vitamin such as vitamin A, be sure to include a little fat in your meal.

Q: **How can I make sure the supplements I'm buying are fresh and fully potent?**

A: There's no way to be absolutely certain. Some supplement labels list expiration dates, indicating the last date on which you should buy or use the product. If you can't find an expiration date, look instead for a product with good outer and inner seals. These seals limit the product's exposure to air.

Q: **How should I store my supplements?**

A: Keep them in opaque containers, not clear ones. And store the containers in a dry, dark place, away from sunlight and heat. Make sure the lids are tightly sealed. Air, sunlight and moisture can degrade the potency of supplements.

DIETARY SOURCES

Q: **Can you remind me which foods are naturally rich in retinol?**

A: Certainly. Liver (including beef, chicken and fish livers) contains a lot of retinol. Fish livers especially rich in retinol are those from cod, halibut, salmon and shark. Butter, egg yolks, cream and whole milk also contain retinol.

Q: What did you say about vitamin A and fats?

A: Vitamin A, or retinol, is best absorbed with fat since it is a fat-soluble vitamin. But since the foods that naturally contain retinol come from animals and are already high in fat, you won't need to add extra fat to satisfy that requirement.

Q: Aren't some foods fortified with vitamin A?

A: Yes. Low-fat milk products and breakfast cereals are among the most common fortified foods, though even candy bar manufacturers are now trying to make their products more nutritious.

Q: What foods are rich in carotenoids?

A: Let's look at the major carotenoids we consume, which are beta carotene, lycopene, lutein and zeaxanthin, alpha carotene, cryptoxanthin and canthaxanthin. Among these, beta carotene, lycopene and lutein are the most abundant. Beta carotene is found in yellow-orange fruits and vegetables and in many green vegetables. Carrots, kale, parsley, spinach, apricots, cantaloupe, dandelion greens, sweet potatoes, fennel, dill, collard greens, peaches, plums, pumpkin, red peppers and watercress are among the richest sources.

For lycopene, all tomato products, fresh tomatoes, scallions, red grapefruits, watermelon, apricots and guava juice are among the richest sources.

The following fruits and vegetables contain high amounts of lycopene: tomato juice and tomato paste (2 milligrams per ounce), watermelon and pink grapefruit (1 milligram per ounce).

For lutein and zeaxanthin, the richest sources are leafy green vegetables, especially kale. Other greens rich in lutein and zeaxanthin include beet greens, celery, chicory, dill, endive, collard greens, mustard greens, parsley, okra, spinach, watercress and Swiss chard. Red peppers contain plenty of both lutein and zeaxanthin as well. Smaller amounts are contained in many other fruits and vegetables, including kiwifruits, cantaloupe, asparagus, broccoli, corn, cabbage, leeks, green peas, pumpkin, brussels sprouts, okra, romaine lettuce and summer squash.

> *The following vegetables contain high amounts of lutein and zeaxanthin: kale (6 milligrams per ounce), collard greens (5 milligrams per ounce), spinach and watercress (4 milligrams per ounce).*

For alpha carotene, pumpkin and carrots are among the richest sources. For cryptoxanthin, oranges and orange juice are common sources, along with peaches, mangoes and nectarines. Red, orange and yellow fruits and vegetables contain canthaxanthin.

Q: Do I need to do anything special to help my body absorb carotenoids?

A: Yes. Research indicates that beta carotene and lycopene may be best absorbed when eaten with a bit of fat, such as the oil-and-vinegar dressing on a salad. And at least two studies suggest that more lycopene is absorbed when the foods containing it are cooked.

Q: Why would cooking make a difference?

A: Some investigators propose that cooking and chopping breaks down sturdy cell walls, making lycopene more accessible. They also point out that cooked tomato products usually include added fat, which would aid absorption.

Q: Is there anything else I should know about preparing foods rich in carotenoids and vitamin A?

A: Yes. Vitamin A and beta carotene can be destroyed by heat, by alkalis such as baking soda, by light and by air. Because beta carotene can be destroyed by exposure to air, carrot juice should be consumed right after being made. Fruits and vegetables are most nutritious when eaten soon after they have been picked.

Q: How quickly will my body benefit if I increase my intake of fruits and vegetables?

A: Apparently, within a matter of days. In a small study, healthy men and women ate a controlled diet with moderate fat and a high carotenoid content for two 15-day periods. Researchers measured blood carotenoid levels before and after each 15-day period and found that blood concentrations of lutein, cryptoxanthin, alpha carotene, beta carotene and lycopene had risen significantly by day six. And those study participants given additional broccoli (a lutein-rich food) had an additional rise in their blood levels of lutein (*American Journal of Clinical Nutrition,* October 1996).

Q: That's good news. How can I be sure to keep learning about the benefits of carotenoids and vitamin A?

A: If you regularly read a daily newspaper, you will be likely to find out about research results considered relevant to large groups of people. This information often makes it to television and radio as well, though usually in a less detailed form. If you're up for a trip to your local library, you can ask at the information desk to see some health and nutrition publications for more nutrition news. If your interest is strong, you may want to subscribe to a health newsletter that addresses your areas of interest and keeps you informed about new findings. And no matter what you do to stay current, remember to eat plenty of fruits and vegetables!

GLOSSARY

Alpha carotene: A carotenoid found most abundantly in carrots and pumpkin.

Alveoli: Tiny air sacs in the lungs.

Antioxidant: A substance with the ability to interfere with oxygen-generated, or oxidative, reactions. Antioxidants can prevent the production of oxidants (free radicals) and neutralize free radicals, preventing or reducing the damage they cause. Some carotenoids, vitamins C and E and selenium are known antioxidants.

Apoptosis: A process that immune system cells use to break down and destroy cells, including tumor cells.

Atherosclerosis: A condition in which the inner layers of the artery walls become thick and irregular due to deposits of fat, cholesterol and other substances.

Basal cell carcinoma: A type of skin cancer that starts in the lowest layer of the epidermis.

Beta carotene: A carotenoid found in some fruits and vegetables, including cantaloupe and carrots. It can be converted to vitamin A by enzymes in the intestinal wall and liver.

B lymphocyte: A white blood cell that triggers the production of antibodies to neutralize potentially harmful substances.

Canthaxanthin: A carotenoid that brings a red pigment to many vegetables and fruits.

Cardiovascular disease: A category of conditions affecting the heart and arteries, including heart attack, congestive heart failure, coronary-artery disease, atherosclerosis and stroke.

Carotenoid: Any of a group of red, yellow or orange pigments that are found in foods such as carrots, cantaloupe, sweet potatoes and leafy green vegetables. The body converts some of these substances to vitamin A.

Cataract: A clouding of the eye's transparent lens that blocks light from reaching the retina, obstructing vision.

Celiac disease: An inherited, chronic allergy to gluten (a protein) that harms digestion and fat absorption, including the absorption of fat-soluble vitamins such as vitamin A.

Chemoprevention trial: A study that tests a substance thought to prevent cancer against a placebo to see if participants taking the substance are less likely to get cancer.

Cholesterol: A white, waxy substance found naturally throughout the body that belongs to a class of compounds called sterols. The body needs cholesterol to make hormones, vitamin D and bile acids and to build cells.

Clinical trial: A study conducted in a medical setting that tries out a treatment with people who have a specific condition that may be helped by the treatment. Study participants are carefully observed for effects.

Coronary-artery disease: A condition in which atherosclerosis occurs in one or more of the coronary arteries, the spaghetti-size arteries that deliver blood to the heart. A heart attack is a symptom of coronary-artery disease.

Cryptoxanthin: A carotenoid found in some fruits and vegetables, including oranges and peaches. It can be converted to vitamin A by enzymes in the intestinal wall and liver.

Cystic fibrosis: A hereditary disease that thickens fluids secreted from many glands, causing inflammation and damage in the lungs and elsewhere. Cystic fibrosis increases the risk of vitamin A and beta carotene deficiencies.

Dietary Reference Intake (DRI): A dietary recommendation made by the National Academy of Sciences. DRIs, which include four categories of reference intakes, are intended to replace the Recommended Dietary Allowances. They include the Recommended Dietary Allowance, Adequate Intake, Estimated Average Requirement and Tolerable Upper Intake Level.

DRI: See **Dietary Reference Intake (DRI)**.

Emphysema: A disease that damages the alveoli, tiny air sacs in the lungs, causing narrowed airways and restricted breathing.

Epidermis: The top layer of the skin.

Epithelial tissue: A kind of tissue that covers surfaces and lines tubes and cavities throughout the body.

Essential mineral: A mineral essential for survival that the body can't produce, making it necessary to take it in through diet and/or supplementation.

Essential vitamin: A vitamin essential for survival that the body can't produce, making it necessary to take it in through diet and/or supplementation.

Fat soluble: Able to be dissolved in fat. Fat-soluble vitamins can be stored in the body for a long time and require some fat for absorption. Vitamin A is fat soluble.

Free radical: The waste product formed when a molecule interacts with oxygen. These molecular fragments, or oxidants, are unbalanced and attempt to steal electrons from other molecules. Free radical damage can be cumulative and has been linked to degenerative diseases such as heart disease, cancer and arthritis.

Immune response: The way the immune system deploys its resources to protect the body from harm.

Immune system: A complex, interactive system that protects the body from disease organisms and other potentially harmful substances.

International unit (I.U.): An arbitrary unit of measurement that allows the various forms of certain vitamins—notably E, A and D—to be compared with one another.

I.U.: See **International unit (I.U.)**.

LDL: See **Low-density lipoprotein (LDL)**.

Lipid peroxidation: The oxidation of fats, or lipids, in the body, including the oxidation of LDL cholesterol. Lipid peroxidation is believed to be the first step in the development of atherosclerosis.

Low-density lipoprotein (LDL): The so-called bad cholesterol that can lead to clogged arteries. High levels of LDL cholesterol have been linked to increased risk of heart disease.

Lutein: A carotenoid found in leafy green vegetables. Together with zeaxanthin, lutein is responsible for the macula's yellowish color.

Lycopene: A carotenoid found in tomato products. Lycopene is a more powerful antioxidant than beta carotene.

Lymphocyte: A white blood cell that is part of the immune system's arsenal. Classes of lymphocytes, which are found in the blood and the lymphatic vessels, include B lymphocytes, T lymphocytes and natural killer cells.

Macula: A tiny yellowish area at the center of the retina believed to have something to do with color vision.

Macular degeneration: The age-related degeneration of the macula; a leading cause of blindness in the elderly.

Megadose: A very large dose. By scientific definition, a megadose is a dose of 10 times the RDA or more.

Melanoma: A cancer that starts in the pigment-producing cells of the skin and can spread quickly through the body.

Mesothelioma: A tumor in the lung that often results from occupational exposure to asbestos. Mesothelioma can be fatal.

Mineral: A nonorganic compound that does not contain carbon and does not originate from living organisms.

Monocyte: A white blood cell that controls some tumor-fighting aspects of immune response.

Natural killer cell: A class of lymphocyte that is a powerful killer of germs and cancer cells from the time it is formed and that controls some activities of B and T lymphocytes and phagocytes.

Night blindness: Difficulty seeing in the dark; an early symptom of vitamin A deficiency.

Nutrient: A substance used by the body that must be supplied from foods consumed. The six classes of nutrients are water, proteins, carbohydrates, fats, minerals and vitamins.

Oral leukoplakia: Smooth, hard, irregular, white patches on the tongue and cheek that often result from smoking. Oral leukoplakia can become cancerous.

Oxidation: A chemical process in which a molecule combines with oxygen, resulting in a change in its molecular structure, such as a loss of electrons, that leads it to become imbalanced. Oxidation produces free radicals, which are believed to play many destructive roles in the body. Antioxidant nutrients such as vitamins C and E help control oxidation.

Phagocyte: A white blood cell that is part of the immune system's arsenal. Phagocytes engulf and digest organisms and cell waste.

Placebo: An inactive substance.

Polyp: A mass of tissue that bulges or projects outward or upward from the normal surface level.

Population study: A study meant to determine the distribution and causes of various health conditions among large groups of people. Data from population studies may serve to focus prevention efforts.

Preformed vitamin A: A term for vitamin A in its complete form as retinol (as opposed to provitamin A).

Promyelocytic leukemia: A life-threatening disease in which immune system cells develop incorrectly and become cancerous, then move through the bloodstream to spread cancer throughout the body.

Pro-oxidant: An agent that increases oxidation, possibly encouraging disease.

Provitamin A: A term for the 60 or so carotenoid precursors of vitamin A.

RDA: See **Recommended Dietary Allowance (RDA)**.

RE: See **Retinol equivalent (RE)**.

Recommended Dietary Allowance (RDA): The level of intake of essential nutrients that, on the basis of scientific knowledge, is judged by the National Academy of Sciences' Food and Nutrition Board to meet the known nutrient needs of practically all healthy people.

Retinoid: Any of about 4,000 substances derived from retinol and created in our bodies and/or in laboratories. As drugs, they successfully treat many skin diseases and some cancers.

Retinol: Vitamin A in its complete form.

Retinol equivalent (RE): A unit of measurement used for retinol and beta carotene to signify the amount of vitamin A provided by either source.

Retinyl palmitate: A water-soluble form of retinol that can be created both in the body and in laboratories.

Rheumatoid arthritis: A chronic disease with inflammatory changes occurring throughout the body's connective tissues.

Squamous cell carcinoma: A type of skin cancer that starts in the middle layer of the epidermis.

Stroke: The sudden loss of function of part of the brain due to an interference in blood supply.

Supplement: A vitamin, mineral or other nutrient taken either alone or in combination to "supplement" the amount received through the diet.

Synthetic retinoid: A derivative of retinol produced in a laboratory.

T lymphocyte: A white blood cell that attacks and kills invaders, produces chemicals that stimulate phagocytes to attack and prompts B lymphocytes to produce antibodies, substances that neutralize harmful invaders such as viruses and bacteria.

Toxicity: The state of being affected by a harmful amount of a substance. Toxicity can result from an accumulation or a single dose of high amounts of vitamin A.

Vitamin: An organic component of food found to be essential in small quantities for normal human metabolism, growth and physical well-being.

Vitamin A: A fat-soluble, clear yellow oil; any of about 4,000 retinoids.

Water soluble: Able to be dissolved in water. The water-soluble vitamins—the B vitamins and vitamin C—are not stored in the body but are quickly excreted.

Zeaxanthin: A carotenoid abundant in leafy green vegetables. Together with zeaxanthin, lutein is responsible for the macula's yellowish color.

INDEX

A

Accutane. *See* Isotretinoin

Acne

isotretinoin effects, 82, 83

tretinoin effects, 82, 83

vitamin A effects, 19, 29, 31

Acneiform dermatosis,
isotretinoin effects, 83

Acute respiratory infection,
vitamin A and children, 38-39

Age, effects, 25, 34-35

Age spots, tretinoin effects, 82

Air pollution, effects, 98

Alcohol, effects, 13, 25, 35,
97, 98

All-trans-retinoic acid,
emphysema, 79-80

Alpha carotene

breast cancer, 51, 53

cardiovascular disease, 67

colorectal cancer, 55

defined, 13, 111

dietary sources, 63, 108-109

prostate cancer, 57

Alveoli, defined, 79, 111

Antioxidants

cardiovascular disease
effects, 20

defined, 20, 22, 111

disease prevention, 34

role of vitamin A, 22, 34

types, 22

Apoptosis, defined, 64, 111

Asbestos-exposed workers,
vitamin A effects, 31, 47, 48

Atherosclerosis

carotenoid effects, 69, 74-76

causes, 74

defined, 68, 111

B

B lymphocytes, defined, 37, 111

Basal cell carcinoma, defined,
59, 111

Beta carotene

breast cancer, 51-54

cancer prevention, 13, 33

cancer risks, 46-50

cancer treatment, 61-62
cardiovascular disease, 65-76
colorectal cancer, 55, 61-62
cystic fibrosis, 78-79, 96
defined, 12, 111
dietary sources, 12-13, 35, 36, 51, 63, 87-88, 96-97, 108-109
drug interactions, 101-102
elderly, 39-41
HIV, 84-86, 101
human papillomavirus (HPV), 40-41
liver cancer, 56
macular degeneration, 82
megadoses
  defined, 100
  effects, 100-101
prostate cancer, 57
rheumatoid arthritis, 84, 87-88
side effects, 28
skin problems, 83-84
sunburn, 83-84
supplement dosage guidelines, 94-95, 96-97
supplement sources, 105
Bile acid sequestrants, effects on vitamin A absorption, 101
Birth control pills
  effects on beta carotene absorption, 101
  retinol level guidelines, 30
Birth defects, retinol levels, 29-30
Bladder cancer, lycopene effects, 43
Blindness. *See* Macular degeneration; Vision

Bone disease, retinol level guidelines, 30
Breast cancer
  beta carotene effects, 51-54
  carotenoid effects, 51-54
  lycopene effects, 43
  vitamin A effects, 50-54, 61

C

Cancer. *See* specific cancer type
Canthaxanthin
  cancer prevention, 64
  defined, 13, 111
  dietary sources, 108-109
  effects, 15, 33
Cardiovascular disease
  beta carotene effects, 13, 49-50, 66-76
  beta carotene supplements, 69-73
  carotenoid effects, 20, 33, 66-76
  defined, 13, 112
  lutein effects, 73, 76
  lycopene effects, 67, 73-75
  prevention, 14, 31, 91
  vitamin A effects, 13, 20, 31, 65-76
  vitamin E effects, 49-50, 66, 70-71
  zeaxanthin effects, 73, 76
Carotenoids. *See also* Alpha carotene; Beta carotene; Canthaxanthin; Cryptoxanthin; Lutein; Lycopene; Zeaxanthin
  absorption guidelines, 109-110
  atherosclerosis, 74-76

blood level studies, 34-36

breast cancer, 51-54

cancer prevention, 41-46, 62-63, 91

cancer treatment, 59-62, 59-65

cardiovascular disease, 65-76, 91

cataracts, 80-81, 91

colorectal cancer, 54-56

common, 13

deficiency, causes, 98

defined, 12, 112

dietary intake studies, 34-36

dietary sources, 14, 25-26, 31, 35, 43, 51, 91, 108-109

drug interactions, 101-102

fat and absorption, 16, 109

fat substitute effects, 102

interaction with other carotenoids, 102

liver cancer, 56

low-density lipoprotein (LDL) oxidation, 74-76

macular degeneration, 81-82, 91

respiratory system, 76-80

rheumatoid arthritis, 84, 87-88, 91

skin cancer prevention, 59

skin problems, 83-84

supplements, 104-105

ultraviolet light exposure, 83

Cataracts

carotenoid effects, 80-81, 91

defined, 80, 112

Celiac disease

defined, 25, 112

vitamin A deficiency, 97

Cervical cancer

beta carotene effects, 50, 61-62

carotenoid effects, 43

lycopene effects, 14

vitamin A effects, 50

Chemoprevention trials, defined, 48-49, 112

Chemotherapy, vitamin A effects, 61, 64

Children

vitamin A deficiency, 97

vitamin A effects, 38-39

Cholesterol, defined, 20, 112

Cholesterol medications

blood carotenoid level reduction, 101-102

effects on vitamin A absorption, 101

Cholestyramine

blood carotenoid level reduction, 101-102

effects on vitamin A absorption, 101

Clinical trial, defined, 32, 112

Cod-liver oil, vitamin A supplement, 104-106

ColBENEMID. *See* Colchicine

Colchicine, effects on beta carotene absorption, 102

Colestid. *See* Colestipol hydrochloride

Colestipol hydrochloride, effects on vitamin A absorption, 101

Colorectal cancer
  beta carotene effects, 41, 61-62
  carotenoid effects, 54-56
  lycopene effects, 52-53, 55
  riboflavin effects, 54
  vitamin A effects, 54-56, 62
  vitamin C effects, 54
Contraceptives, oral
  effects on beta carotene
    absorption, 101
  retinol level guidelines, 30
Coronary-artery disease,
    defined, 74, 112
Cryptoxanthin
  defined, 13, 112
  dietary sources, 108-109
  effects, 33
  human papillomavirus (HPV),
    40
  prostate cancer, 57
Cystic fibrosis
  beta carotene effects, 78-79, 96
  defined, 25, 78, 112
  vitamin A deficiency, 97
  vitamin A effects, 25, 31

D
Dialysis, retinol level guidelines,
    30
Dietary Reference Intakes
    (DRIs), defined, 27, 95, 113
Digestive tract cancer, lycopene
    effects, 14, 57
Dosage guidelines
  beta carotene, 94-95, 96-97
  retinol, 94, 95
  vitamin A, 92-97

DRIs
  defined, 27, 95, 113
  vitamin A, 95
Drug interactions
  carotenoids, 101-102
  vitamin A, 101-102

E
Elderly
  beta carotene effects, 39-41
  vitamin A deficiencies, 25,
    34-35, 97
  vitamin A effects, 39
Emphysema
  defined, 76, 79-80, 113
  retinoid effects, 76, 79-80
Endometrial cancer, prevention,
    43, 50
Epidermis, defined, 58, 113
Epithelial tissue, defined,
    18, 113
Essential minerals, defined,
    22, 113
Essential vitamins, defined,
    22, 113
Etretrinate, psoriasis, 83
Exercise, effects, 98

F
Fat, vitamin A absorption,
    16-17, 109
Fat soluble, defined, 16, 113
Fat substitutes, effects on
    blood carotene levels, 102
Fortified food, vitamin A, 108
Free radicals, defined, 21, 113

G

Gender. *See also* Women

  dosage guidelines, 24, 94, 99

  effects, 34-35

Gout treatment, effects on beta carotene absorption, 102

H

Heart attack

  carotenoid effects, 66-67

  causes, 68

Heart disease. *See* Cardio-vascular disease; Heart attack

HIV

  beta carotene effects, 84-86, 101

  vitamin A effects, 84-86

Human immunodeficiency virus. *See* HIV

Human papillomavirus (HPV), beta carotene effects, 40-41

I

Immune response, defined, 22, 37-38, 113

Immune system

  defined, 19, 36-37, 113

  vitamin A effects, 19, 31, 37-40, 63

Infants, premature, vitamin A effects, 39

International unit (I.U.), defined, 24, 114

Isotretinoin

  acne, 82

  acneiform dermatosis, 83

contraindications, 30

effects, 19, 59, 60

rosacea, 83

seborrheic dermatitis, 83

side effects, 100

vitamin A toxicity, 101

I.U.

  defined, 24, 93, 114

  equivalent for RDA, 94

  supplement measurement guidelines, 106

K

Kidney failure, retinol level guidelines, 30

L

Laxatives, mineral oil, effects on vitamin A absorption, 101

LDL. *See* Low-density lipoprotein (LDL)

Lipid peroxidation, defined, 21, 114

Liver, role in vitamin A storage, 11

Liver cancer

  beta carotene effects, 56

  carotenoid effects, 56

  lycopene effects, 56

  vitamin A effects, 56, 60

Liver disease, retinol level guidelines, 30

Low-density lipoprotein (LDL)

  defined, 68, 114

  oxidation and carotenoids, 74-76

Lung cancer
  beta carotene effects, 43,
    44-46
  risks, beta carotene effects,
    46-50
  treatment, vitamin A effects,
    60-61
Lutein
  breast cancer, 51, 53-54
  cancer prevention, 33
  cardiovascular disease, 73, 76
  cataracts, 80-81
  colorectal cancer, 52-53, 55
  defined, 13, 114
  dietary sources, 14-15, 81,
    108-109
  human papillomavirus (HPV),
    40
  macular degeneration, 14-15,
    81
  prostate cancer, 57
  supplements, 105
Lycopene
  absorption guidelines, 109
  breast cancer, 52
  cancer prevention, 14, 65
  cardiovascular disease, 14, 67,
    73-75
  colorectal cancer, 52-53, 55
  deficiency causes, 98
  defined, 13, 114
  dietary sources, 14, 52, 57-58,
    63, 108-109
  drug interactions, 101-102
  liver cancer, 56
  prostate cancer, 56-58
  supplements, 105

Lymphocytes
  B, defined, 37, 111
  defined, 37, 114
  T, defined, 37, 117

M
Macula, defined, 15, 114
Macular degeneration
  beta carotene effects, 82
  carotenoid effects, 81-82, 91
  defined, 14, 114
Megadoses, defined, 99, 114
Melanoma
  defined, 43, 114
  vitamin A effects, 43, 60
Mesothelioma, defined, 50, 114
Mineral oil laxatives, effects on
    vitamin A absorption, 101
Minerals
  defined, 22, 114
  essential, defined, 22, 113
Monocytes, defined, 41, 115
Multivitamins, content, 26,
    103-104

N
Natural killer cells, defined,
    37, 115
Night blindness
  causes, 80
  defined, 24, 115
Nutrient, defined, 11, 115

O
Olean. *See* Fat substitutes
Olestra. *See* Fat substitutes

Oral leukoplakia, defined, 60, 115

Oxidation, defined, 20-22, 115

P

Palm carotenes

colorectal cancer, 55

defined, 55

Pancreatic cancer, lycopene effects, 57

Phagocytes, defined, 37, 115

Placebo, defined, 38, 115

Polyprenoic acid, effects, 60

Polyps, defined, 54, 115

Population studies, defined, 20, 115

Preformed vitamin A, defined, 11, 115

Pregnancy

retinol contraindications, 29-30

vitamin A effects on HIV transmission, 84-85

Premature infants, vitamin A effects, 88

Pro-oxidant, defined, 49, 116

Probucol, blood carotenoid level reduction, 101-102

Promyelocytic leukemia, defined, 60, 115

Prostate cancer

alpha carotene effects, 57

beta carotene effects, 57

cryptoxanthin effects, 57

lutein effects, 57

lycopene effects, 14, 56-58

risk, vitamin A effects, 56-58

Provitamin A, defined, 11, 116

Psoriasis, etretrinate, 83

Q

Questran. *See* Cholestyramine

R

RDAs

defined, 23, 116

dosage guidelines, 92-93

I.U. equivalent, 94

revised, 27-28, 95

supplement measurement guidelines, 106

RE

defined, 23, 93, 116

dosage guidelines, 92-93

supplement measurement guidelines, 106

Recommended Dietary Allowance (RDA), defined, 23, 116

Rectal cancer, carotenoid effects, 43

Renova. *See* Tretinoin

Respiratory system

carotenoid effects, 76-80

vitamin A effects, 76

Retin-A. *See* Tretinoin

Retinoids

cancer prevention, 44-46, 51

cancer risks, 46-50

defined, 18-19, 43, 116

emphysema, 76, 79-80

skin cancer prevention, 58-59

skin problems, 82-83

synthetic, defined, 19, 116

Retinol
  contraindications, 29-30
  defined, 11, 116
  dietary sources, 26, 107-108
  dosage guidelines, 94, 95
  excessive intake signs, 29
  side effects, 29
Retinol equivalent (RE),
  defined, 23, 116
Retinyl palmitate, defined, 104,
  116
Rheumatoid arthritis, carotenoid
  effects, 84, 87-88, 91
Riboflavin, colorectal cancer,
  54
Rosacea, isotretinoin effects,
  83

S
Seborrheic dermatitis,
  isotretinoin effects, 83
Selenium, antioxidant role, 22
Skin cancer
  beta carotene effects, 64
  vitamin A effects, 19, 43,
    58-59, 60
Skin problems. *See also* Acne;
  Wrinkles
  beta carotene effects, 83-84
  carotenoid effects, 83-84
  ultraviolet light exposure,
    carotenoid effects, 83
  vitamin A effects, 19, 31
Smoking
  effects, 13, 35, 60, 70, 72-73,
    77, 98
  vitamin A effects, 31, 46-48,
    60

Squamous cell carcinoma,
  defined, 58, 116
Stomach cancer
  beta carotene effects, 64
  lycopene effects, 57
Stroke
  causes, 68, 74
  defined, 20, 116
Sunburn, beta carotene effects,
  83-84
Sunscreen, effects, 83-84
Supplements
  absorption guidelines,
    106-107
  beta carotene, 105
  cardiovascular disease,
    69-73
  carotenoid, 104-105
  contraindications, 13, 27
  defined, 13, 116
  expiration, 107
  lutein, 105
  lycopene, 105
  measurement guidelines, 106
  mineral, 103-104
  multivitamin, 26, 103-104
  natural, 105
  side effects, 28
  storage, 107
  store brand vs. brand-name,
    106
  synthetic, 105
  types, 103
  U.S.P. standards, 106-107
Synthetic retinoids, defined,
  19, 116

T

T lymphocytes, defined, 37, 117

Tegison. *See* Etretrinate

Toxicity, defined, 17, 117

Tretinoin

acne, 82

age spots, 82

effects, 19

wrinkles, 82

V

Vision. *See also* Macular degeneration; Night blindness

beta carotene effects, 82

vitamin A effects, 14, 18, 19, 31

Vitamin, defined, 11, 117

Vitamin A. *See also* Beta carotene; Carotenoids; Retinoids; Retinol; Supplements

absorption guidelines, 109-110

breast cancer, 50-54

cancer in women, 50-54

cancer treatment, 59-62, 59-65

cardiovascular disease, 13, 20, 31, 65-76

chemotherapy, 61, 64

children, 38-39

colorectal cancer, 54-56

cystic fibrosis, 25, 31

deficiency

causes, 25, 34-35, 97

signs, 24-25, 97

defined, 11, 117

dietary sources, 11, 12, 25-26, 50-51, 58

effects of different, 15-16

fortified food, 108

dosage guidelines, 92-97

drug interactions, 101-102

effects, 14, 18, 31-33

elderly, 25, 34-35, 39, 97

excess, 16, 17

fat and absorption, 16, 109

HIV, 84-86

immune system, 37-38, 38-40, 63

interaction with vitamin E, 102

interaction with zinc, 102

I.U. guidelines, 24

liver cancer, 56

multivitamins, 26

nutrient interactions, 102

preformed, defined, 11, 115

premature infants, 88

pro-, defined, 11, 116

prostate cancer, 56-58

RDA guidelines, 24

RE guidelines, 24

respiratory system, 76-80

side effects, 28

toxicity

causes, 96

drug interactions, 101

effects, 99

signs, 99-100

vision, 14, 18, 19, 31, 80-82

Vitamin C
  antioxidant role, 22
  colorectal cancer, 54
  lung cancer, 44-45
Vitamin E
  antioxidant role, 22
  cancer in women, 49-50
  cardiovascular disease, 66,
    70-71
  colorectal cancer, 55
  human papillomavirus (HPV),
    40
  lung cancer, 44-45, 46
  vitamin A interaction, 102
Vitamins, essential, defined,
  22, 113

W

Water soluble, defined, 17, 117
Water-soluble vitamins, types, 17
Women. *See also* Gender
  carotenoid effects, 66
  vitamin A effects, 50-54, 66
  vitamin E effects, 49-50
Wrinkles, tretinoin effects, 82

Z

Zeaxanthin
  breast cancer, 51, 53
  cardiovascular disease, 73-76
  cataracts, 80-81
  defined, 13, 117
  dietary sources, 14-15, 81,
    108-109
  macular degeneration, 14-15,
    81
Zinc, vitamin A interaction, 102